Losing Weight
When
Diets Fail

Losing Weight When Diets Fail

The Clinically Proven Power Programming
Method for Amazingly Easy,
Fail-Proof, Diet-Free Weight Loss

TOM KERSTING, PH.D.

HARBOR PRESS
GIG HARBOR, WA

Library of Congress Cataloging-in-Publication Data
Kersting, Tom, 1972–
    Losing weight when diets fail: the clinically proven Power Programming method for amazingly easy, fail-proof, diet-free weight loss/Tom Kersting.
    p. cm.
    Includes index.
    ISBN-13: 978-0-936197-52-4
    ISBN-10: 0-936197-52-8
1. Weight loss. 2. Reducing diets. 3. Weight loss—Psychological aspects. I. Title.
RM222.2.K47 2007
613.2'5—dc22   2006043488

IMPORTANT NOTICE

The ideas, positions, and statements in this book can have an impact on your health, may not be suitable for everyone, and may in some cases conflict with orthodox, mainstream medical opinion. Do not attempt self-diagnosis, and do not embark upon any kind of self-treatment or dietary or exercise program without qualified medical supervision. Nothing in this book should be construed as a promise of benefits or of results to be achieved, or a guarantee by the author or publisher of the safety or efficacy of its contents. The author, the publisher, its editors, and its employees disclaim any liability, loss, or risk incurred directly or indirectly as a result of the use or application of any of the contents of this book. If you are not willing to be bound by this disclaimer, please return your copy of the book to the publisher for a full refund.

LOSING WEIGHT WHEN DIETS FAIL
The Clinically Proven Power Programming Method for Amazingly Easy, Fail-Proof, Diet-Free Weight Loss

Printed in the United States of America.

10 9 8 7 6 5 4 3 2 1

Harbor Press and the Nautilus shell logo are registered trademarks of Harbor Press, Inc.

Harbor Press, Inc.
P.O. Box 1656
Gig Harbor, WA 98335

www.harborpress.com

*For my wonderful wife, Krista, who has been
there with me every step of the way, not just
during the daunting task of writing a book, but in
every endeavor I pursue. You are encouraging and
inspirational, a wonderful wife, a friend and a
special mother to our children. The moment I laid eyes
on you I knew I wanted to spend the rest of my
life with you. Your hard work throughout your life
is what sparked the flame in me to pursue
my dreams. I love you, Krista.*

Visit Dr. Kersting on the Internet at

www.losingweightwhendietsfail.com
and
www.harborpress.com

Contents

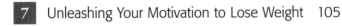

Preface

When I was in college, baseball was my life. It was my dream, my passion. I was one of the starting pitchers on my team and, more than anything else in the world, I wanted to be a great pitcher. But something started to go wrong during my second season. I began to lose control of my pitches and of my mind. Every time I went out on the mound I froze. It felt as if my pitching skills had just evaporated. And then, it happened. . .

It was the first inning of an important game and I was the starting pitcher. My nerves began to take over and my confidence was going downhill by the minute. The pressure was intense. Sure enough, I loaded the bases on twelve straight pitches. I wasn't able to throw one single strike! This was not Little League baseball; you just don't do that at this level. Finally, my coach took me out of the game. I was devastated and demoralized.

I thought I was finished with baseball, washed up for good, until a teammate of mine suggested that I see a psychologist who specializes in sports-related problems. When I visited him, it literally transformed my life. Not only did the psychologist help me become a much better pitcher, he showed me that I could use the amazing power of my mind to change my behavior in virtually any situation in my life.

The technique he used was surprisingly simple and basic, but more effective than I had ever thought possible. I began by lying down on the couch in his office with soothing music playing in the background. He asked me to close my eyes and he began talking to me in a soothing, relaxing tone. As he continued to speak I became deeply relaxed. Then he asked me to imagine myself on the pitcher's mound, feeling confident and intensely focused on the catcher's glove.

With my mind in this calm and relaxed state he told me that all I had to do was breathe deeply and count down from 10 to 1 every time I took the mound. He said I would feel relaxed, confident, and focused and I would be successful. When the session was over I wondered how this was going to help me. It seemed way too simple and almost silly. Fortunately, nothing could have been further from the truth.

Not only did this session and two follow-up visits help me with my pitching, it changed my life completely. I went on to a successful college career in baseball, but more importantly I developed a special confidence in myself, knowing that the incredible power to change my behavior and my life was within my own mind. In fact, this "miracle cure" fascinated me so much and had such a tremendous effect on my life, I decided to give up baseball and pursue a career in psychology.

After college, while I was in graduate school studying psychology and human development, I became less active physically and started gaining weight—more than 20 pounds. I wasn't feeling good about myself and I knew I had to go on some kind of diet. I did what most people do to lose weight: bought a treadmill, gave-up soda, and started watching my calories. I'd run on the treadmill for a few weeks, stop for a few months, drink soda for a few weeks and stop for a few weeks, eat McDonald's, not eat McDonald's. There was no consistency to my behavior. It frustrated me. And I wasn't losing the weight!

Then it hit me. Why couldn't I use the same mind techniques to lose weight that I had used years before to improve my pitching? I took what I learned from my psychology courses and my sessions with the sports psychologist and created my own mental weight loss program. I discovered that the best way to think about the mind when you're trying to change behavior is to compare it to a computer. All you need to do to lose weight quickly and easily is reprogram your mental computer with new weight loss software. That's why I call my new approach *Power Programming*.

I began with the same basic techniques I had learned and then took them to another level. Rather than just imagining myself feeling confident and in control of my behavior, which is what I had done to improve my pitching, I intensified the images in my mind by accessing all of my senses. In other words, I created powerful new software to program into my mental computer. For example, I imagined chewing on delicious, mouth-watering fruit, while having no desire for desserts and sweets. I focused on the wonderful feeling I get after a long run—the "runner's high." I saw myself sitting down at my favorite restaurant eating slowly, savoring the flavors and enjoying my meal more than ever before. I imagined myself leaving food on my plate and feeling empowered every time I did it. The more creative I became, the more readily these images and messages began to carry over into real life. I realized how effectively the mind can transform long-term, automatic behaviors when you use the power of your mind to its greatest potential.

Not only did I find myself eating less, eating healthier foods, and exercising religiously, I did it all effortlessly and without resistance. The struggle to control my cravings and my weight disappeared, and losing weight became automatic and natural.

Well, that was nine years and 20 pounds ago, and I haven't stopped since. The best part is that I've been able to share my Power Programming techniques with thousands of my clients over the years, and almost all of them have permanently lost weight using my program.

Now I'm in the best shape of my life, and I attribute every bit of it to my mind. Every day I get up early and exercise, I avoid desserts like the plague, and all of it is absolutely effortless. I haven't touched a soda in years and I love drinking water. I don't go anywhere near fried foods or fast-food restaurants. I love my life. I love my self-control. I love my self-esteem. I love having energy. I love looking in the mirror. I love believing in myself. And I love helping others do the same. Whether you need to lose 10 pounds or 100 pounds, whether you can exercise three days a week or every day, this program can work for you. So, dig in and get ready to crack the code to your own weight loss computer. Before you know it, you'll eliminate excess weight, keep it off for good, and finally live the life you deserve!

Acknowledgments

My dear editor, Debby Young, where do I begin? I thank you from the bottom of my heart for taking a chance with me and this work. Without you, this book would not have happened. You have become a real friend, someone I can trust and lean on. Your effort toward this book is of an old-fashioned sort, combining the soft stroke of Joe Torre with the fire of Tiger Woods. You pushed me to work my hardest and you did it in such a soft, encouraging way. I cannot thank you enough, Debby.

I'd like to thank Harry Lynn, my publisher. You believed in me and took a chance, not something every publisher is willing to do with a first-time author. Your patience for perfection cannot be matched. You helped make this book what it is. Thank you, Harry, thank you.

I want to thank my wonderful wife Krista and my little boy Matthew and baby daughter Ashlyn. You are the air I breathe. You are my rock. You are my life. I love you both more than anything in this world and I thank you for putting up with me during this arduous task we call publishing.

I want to thank my parents, Marge and Joe. The values, integrity, spirituality and love you have given to me throughout my life have made me the person I am. You've made me believe in myself since the day I was born. I love you both very much.

I want to thank Carrie, Peggy and Joey, my sisters and brother and my best friends. I am the luckiest man in the world to have shared my childhood and adulthood with all of you. You epitomize the word family and I love you dearly.

And I want to thank the Lord above for everything I have been blessed with, for giving me the opportunity to live a special life and to help others find themselves.

Introduction

Whether it's the grapefruit diet or the rice diet, the Atkins diet, the Weight Watchers plan, low carbs, no carbs, or lots of carbs, it seems as if everybody is trying to lose weight. Unfortunately, most just aren't successful, and those who do manage to lose 10 or 15 pounds inevitably put it all back on again the minute they stop dieting. The bottom line is that Americans are getting fatter and less healthy as they spend more money and time than ever before trying to get thin.

Clearly, we're a nation in desperate need of a weight loss strategy that works. But most people think that losing weight means struggling hard and sweating off every single pound. It's true that traditional diets are all about denying yourself, feeling hungry all the time, and being miserable. That's what stops a lot of people from even beginning a diet, and it's why so many others who do go on a diet eventually revert to their old habits.

The amazing truth is that weight loss doesn't have to involve struggle, nor does it have to be difficult and expensive. There's a way to make unwanted pounds disappear more easily than you ever thought possible, without having to buy fancy equipment or truckloads of special food.

You undoubtedly know that the key to losing weight is to eat less and exercise more. But what you might not realize is that losing weight will be an uphill struggle so long as you don't change your *subconscious* approach to eating and exercising. Unless you erase and replace your subconscious behavior patterns, you'll end up sabotaging yourself every time.

In this book, you'll learn the simple, powerful, and effective way to make pounds vanish without struggle and effort, and it doesn't have anything to do with measuring, counting calories, or looking up the glycemic indexes of hundreds of different foods. The truth is this: *the power to control your weight lies within your subconscious mind.* Once you learn how to tap into and use your subconscious mind, you'll find yourself losing weight faster than you ever thought possible. You'll prove to yourself that losing weight is easy and effortless. And best of all, you'll *keep* the weight off!

I call this simple yet incredible technique *Power Programming,* and it's helped thousands of my clients lose weight quickly, effortlessly, and permanently. The truth is, Power Programming can be used for all sorts of reasons other than weight loss: to change a habit, eliminate a phobia or anxiety, heal the mind or body, or improve study skills, creative abilities, or sports performance. This book and the Power Programming CD that comes with it will show you how to rid yourself of excess weight forever, without struggle and effort! When you read this book, you'll read about lots of people just like yourself, who used Power Programming techniques to make excess weight vanish, almost like magic.

The best way to understand how Power Programming works is to think of your mind as a powerful computer. Right now, your mental computer—your subconscious mind—is filled with obsolete, virus-infected software that causes you to eat when you're not really hungry, binge when you're unhappy, lonely, or frustrated, and dive into high-calorie comfort foods when cravings strike. The good news is that you can use Power Programming to uninstall these make-me-fat programs and viruses and replace them with effective new make-me-thin software. Cravings will vanish and good eating and exercise habits will be automatically ingrained in your everyday behavior patterns. It's as simple as that! Power Programming will give you the tools and insight you need to reprogram your mental computer and fat-proof yourself once and for all.

Your book comes with a bound-in audio CD containing three complete Power Programming sessions and additional conditioning exercises. But please resist the temptation to open the CD and begin listening before you've read the book. You'll benefit much more from the Power Programming sessions on the CD, losing more weight than you ever thought possible, if you finish reading the book first. It will tell you how and why Power Programming works so effectively while weight loss diets fail. And it will start you down the road to a lifetime of healthy eating and exercise without struggle or self-denial.

In Part One of this book I'll explain exactly what Power Programming is. I'll zero in on the real reasons you eat heaping portions of food, snack on high calorie sweets, or eat yourself into a coma. You'll also discover why dieting is almost always fated to fail. You'll learn how to unlock the power of your subconscious mind, gaining a whole new awareness that will cause you to say to yourself, "Ahh, now I get it." Part One ends with healthy eating strategies and meal menus which, when coupled with your Power Programming weight loss techniques, will cause you to enjoy every minute of growing thin.

Part Two describes clearly and simply how you can use the power of your mind to take control of your eating. I'm not talking about "willing" yourself to control your eating. That's dieting. That's using your *conscious* mind—an approach which almost always fails in the long run. I'm talking about enlisting the power of your *subconscious* mind, your mental computer, the real control center for your actions. I'll introduce you to relaxation, imagery, and suggestion techniques—the passwords that will give you access to your subconscious supercomputer. Remember, your subconscious mind is a powerful computer, just waiting for you to program in behavior patterns that will rid you of excess weight for the rest of your life.

By the time you get to Part Three, you'll have the understanding you need to move on to the final and most important phase of my weight loss program. In Part Three I'll explain how to use your Power Programming CD to uninstall the mental programming that's making you overweight. And I'll show you how to reprogram your subconscious to achieve your perfect weight with glowing health and enough energy for two persons.

Your CD provides you with three easy-to-use Power Programming sessions—some of the same ones that have produced amazing results for the clients I see in my practice. Each session is designed to be used for one week initially. In other words, you'll listen to the first session every day for the first week; then you'll listen to the second session every day for the second week; and, finally, you'll listen to the third session every day for the third and final week. You should see excess weight starting to melt away during the very first week. Within three short weeks, after having listened to all three sessions, you'll be solidly on track for achieving your weight loss goals!

Remember, once you download the new software on your CD and reboot your mental computer, you'll lose weight automatically, and you'll never have to diet again. Power Programming will allow you to slice right through cravings, compulsions, and dangerous eating habits. You'll lose weight without a struggle and you'll gain the motivation you need to make it last a lifetime.

This book includes two special features. First, at the end of most chapters, you'll find a simple weight loss activity such as a short quiz or a warm-up exercise that will help you reinforce the ideas covered in the chapter you've just read and will prepare you for the Power Programming CD. Second, it provides you with Power Programming scripts you can record and use at home after tailoring them to your own individual needs. Recording your own customized scripts is purely optional. But it can be a useful tool for anyone who wants more variety, or who wants to target and overcome specific stumbling blocks.

But right now, let's move on to Chapter 1 where I'll tell you exactly what Power Programming is and how it can completely transform your life.

PART ONE

Power Programming
Your Weight Loss
Computer

THE MAGIC OF
POWER PROGRAMMING

Power Programming is unlike any weight loss program you've ever tried. Get ready to say goodbye to dieting, cravings, and guilt. Be prepared to swing open the doors to your mind and flip on a high-voltage switch that is so strong, so automatic, that not even grandma's Thanksgiving apple cobbler will tempt you.

Power Programming is simple. It's all about using your mind's natural ability to change your behavior without struggle or effort. Through Power Programming, you'll enter the vast universe of your subconscious mind and you'll "reprogram" it however you wish. If you want to hit the delete key and end unhealthy cravings for good, you'll succeed. If you want to pump yourself up with a high-speed burst of motivation that will get you to exercise on a regular basis, you will. Once you apply my Power Programming techniques, you won't need to search for answers anymore. Your subconscious mind will do it for you naturally.

Here's how Dawn Power Programmed her mind to accomplish her weight loss goals:

> Dawn was 42 years old with a high-powered job and a major weight problem. Like many people I meet, she was desperate to lose weight, but skeptical about my Power Programming techniques. However, once she had reached a point of desperation, she was willing to try just about anything. She had been through all of the fad diets already, and she was never able to stick to them. Dawn explained to me that every

time she dieted, she felt even more miserable than she was before she began.

During our initial consultation, the reason for Dawn's weight gain became clear. In fact, she knew all along what it was, but she just didn't know how to stop it. She snacked a lot between meals, always finished everything on her plate, and never exercised. Although she tried to correct these habits when she was dieting, it never worked. She always returned to her old habits because changing was just too much of a struggle. Because of my training and experience, it was obvious to me that her habits were entirely subconscious.

Using Power Programming, Dawn was able to reprogram her subconscious mind so that she wanted to eat less, to avoid snacks, and to exercise regularly. In fact, it became easy for her to do all three! As soon as she began, the pounds started to melt away. Dawn was able to lose 45 pounds, and since then she's succeeded in keeping it off without sticking to a diet. She says that Power Programming worked for her unlike any diet she had ever tried. Now Dawn's dieting days are over for good. She looks great and she feels terrific about herself!

Before you can achieve the same success that Dawn did, you need to understand how your mind actually influences your behavior.

POWER PROGRAMMING MADE EASY

If you're like Dawn, you're probably feeling at least a little skeptical about Power Programming. It just sounds too good to be true. How can something that seems so much like magic actually work? Before you can learn the answers to these questions, first you need to understand some basic things about the mind and the way it works.

Think of your mind as a computer. The hard drive of the computer—the part that stores all of the programming you will use—is your *subconscious* mind. It's the part of your mind that controls, among many other things, your eating habits, your compulsions, your cravings, and your self-control. Right now, your mental hard drive is loaded with software that is causing you to overeat and make unhealthy food choices. To change that and reverse the bad habits, all you need to do is uninstall the old software and reinstall new weight loss software that will help you lose pounds without even trying. This is exactly what Power Programming is designed to do. It makes it possible for you to reprogram your mental computer with new software that will make your weight loss problems a thing of the past. With Power Programming you can transform your subconscious mind, take weight off and keep it off permanently.

Let me make it clear that there's no hocus-pocus in Power Programming. It actually involves a very natural process that you experience every day: bringing your mind to a different level of consciousness, a level that is ultra-receptive to new ideas and behaviors. This ultra-receptive level is your subconscious mind, and it controls all of your behavior, although you don't realize it as it's happening. Everyone has the ability to access his or her subconscious mind. In fact, you do it every day without even giving it much thought. Here are some examples of what I mean:

Whenever you daydream, you enter an altered state of consciousness. Anytime your mind drifts and wanders, anytime you're exposed to images in a movie or on TV, anytime you're focused on reading, and right before you fall asleep, you enter different levels of consciousness. When you're curled up securely on your couch under a warm blanket, deeply engrossed in a suspenseful novel, you are temporarily detached from your conscious world and very much submerged in your subconscious world. If you've ever jumped out of your seat in fright during a movie, you were experiencing some form of a subconscious state. In fact, at this very moment, as you're reading this book, your mind has distanced itself from conscious awareness. It has entered a shallow level of subconscious activity and if you kept going to the next level, deep within your subconscious, your mind would be ripe for Power Programming.

You're Always in Control

Every so often, someone will ask me if they will lose control of their ability to make decisions and exercise judgments while being in this altered state of consciousness. I'd like to clear that up now. Whenever you are in a subconscious state, you actually have more control. For example, if you are practicing Power Programming techniques at home and a fire breaks out, you will open your eyes and run to safety. You won't lie there, paralyzed, unable to escape. And you won't somehow get "stuck" in a subconscious state of mind. At any time you want to, all you have to do is open your eyes.

If you are driving along in your car and a deer jumps in front of you, will you hit the deer and keep on driving in dreamy oblivion without realizing what has happened? Of course not! Your instincts will kick in, you'll instantly "wake up" and return to conscious awareness, and you'll do everything possible to avoid hitting the deer. When using Power Programming, the same self-control applies. At any time you want to, you can open your eyes and return to normal consciousness.

Four States of Consciousness

Most people don't realize that their consciousness changes from moment to moment. In fact, your mind moves through four different states of consciousness every day: *beta, theta, alpha* and *delta.*

- *Beta* is the waking state, when your brain waves are moving the fastest. This is when your conscious mind is involved in logical thought.
- *Alpha* is the prime state for Power Programming. It is a "half-awake" state, when your mind is relaxed, distanced from conscious activity. Brain waves in alpha are slower than in beta. As you start to drift into sleep at night and just as you wake up, you're in the alpha state. You sink into deep relaxation during alpha, and your subconscious opens up to become receptive to new stimuli.

■ **Theta** is the "dreaming" state, when your brain wave activity starts to slow down even more. You experience extreme relaxation and conscious separation along with deep, dreamy thoughts, and you may be unaware of your physical body. Some people can reach theta levels during Power Programming.

■ **Delta** is the deep sleep state. Brain wave activity is slowest during delta. Power Programming cannot occur when you are in the delta state.

Every night when you go to bed, you slowly move through all four of these states of consciousness. As you climb into bed, you're in a beta state. Then as you curl up and close your eyes, you move through alpha into theta. Finally, when you are fast asleep, you enter the delta state. In order to wake up and return to beta, you must pass through all four states again. This means that every day you experience levels of consciousness that are conducive to Power Programming.

"Okay," you say, "so my mind wanders and drifts every day. What does that have to do with losing weight?"

Everything. It's the key to losing weight more effortlessly than you ever thought possible.

THE POWER OF YOUR SUBCONSCIOUS MIND

Everything you do starts with a thought: walking the dog, reading a book, eating a double bacon cheeseburger for lunch. But there are two kinds of thoughts: conscious and subconscious. Whenever something "comes to mind," it is a conscious thought. Unintended thoughts (those that come to you out of the blue) come from the subconscious. As long as thoughts remain deeply buried in the subconscious and don't come to the surface, you're unaware of them. But these are the very thoughts that determine most of our actions. Although most of the events you experienced in life are consciously forgotten, they are never forgotten in your subconscious. Yet they do influence your actions, beliefs, and feelings. For example, if you're afraid of spiders, at one time in your life you may have been exposed to a frightening situation involving spiders. Although your conscious mind might not recall the incident, your subconscious mind will always remember it. So, if you *consciously* try to overcome your fear of spiders, it won't work, because your conscious mind doesn't remember how the fear came about. It just knows that it's afraid. Similarly, if you compulsively reach for food when you're feeling stressed or unhappy, you don't know why. All you know is that the ice cream you're spooning into your mouth gives you comfort. The underlying reason—the programming—that triggers eating when you are stressed is buried deep inside your subconscious. And this behavior pattern will continue until you wipe the slate clean and reprogram your subconscious mind.

Your subconscious mind is a memory storehouse, similar to the hard drive in your computer, a place where everything that you have ever experienced is recorded. Every time you savor the crunchy, salty taste of a potato chip, every time you salivate over a TV cooking program, every time you groan with ecstasy while making a bowl of ice cream disappear, the experience is imprinted in your mental computer's memory.

The accumulated power of these experiences profoundly influences your behaviors. If you just can't put down that bag of potato chips, get out of bed to exercise, or stop eating every bite of food on your plate, it's because your mental computer is programmed to make you do all of these things—the very things that make you gain weight.

With my Power Programming techniques you can turn the process around. You can wipe your mental hard drive clean and install brand new software that will cause you to do the very things that make you *lose* weight. For example, here's how Mary Power Programmed her subconscious mind for a whole new attitude toward exercise:

Mary was 200 pounds overweight and desperate. Like many people, she'd tried just about every diet and failed in the end. When she came to me for Power Programming, the most important goal for her was to begin exercising. She lived in a condominium community with a beautiful fitness center, but to her, exercising seemed torturous, and she couldn't bear the thought of getting up in the morning to do it. She was also insecure about what people at the fitness center would think about her because she was so overweight.

During our first Power Programming session, Mary easily relaxed and drifted off into a subconscious state of mind. Then, I guided her through a powerful mental scene. She imagined herself walking confidently out of her condo and going directly to the fitness center with her head held high. She felt strong, motivated, and in control during this scene. She not only was motivated to get on the treadmill, she enjoyed every minute of it. Finally, I suggested that her first waking thought each morning would be to exercise, and that she'd feel eager and determined to get out of bed.

When she returned the following week, she told me that she woke up two or three times every night with a burning desire to exercise. She felt excited, the way a kid feels the night before Christmas. Mary used the treadmill six out of seven days that week and did it without a struggle. She looked forward to it so much, it became a part of her daily routine, one that she's continued to this very day. Through Power Programming, she conditioned her subconscious mind to believe that exercise is desirable and fun. Mary eventually lost 125 pounds and today she's in the best shape, both mentally and physically, of her whole life.

With my Power Programming techniques, Mary was able to transform her subconscious attitude toward exercise. Instead of associating exercise with struggle, she now associates it with fun and excitement. With simple reprogramming techniques, she was able to transform her weight—and her life.

Images and Suggestion Become Reality

If you've ever seen the movie *Rocky*, you know it can trigger intense feelings of determination. *Casablanca, Bambi,* or *Old Yeller* may have moved you to tears. *The Shining* probably sent shivers down your back. But if you really think about it, you're reacting to images on a movie screen, not real life. These images aren't real, and yet you respond as if they were. Did you ever stop to wonder how a few words on a page, or an image in a movie, can make you laugh out loud, or cry, or gasp, or giggle?

When you mentally separate yourself from your conscious surroundings, and you relax and become encapsulated in a dreamy subconscious world, you become hypersensitive to images and suggestions and you naturally react to them. You don't think about it; you just react. This is how your subconscious mind operates.

When you deliberately induce this kind of dreamy hypersensitivity, you tap into your subconscious and become receptive to what I call Power Programming. By making positive suggestions to yourself during Power Programming, you harness the incredible power of your subconscious to change your behavior. If those suggestions target your eating and exercise habits, you're going to be able to change your weight without even thinking about it.

Sound crazy? Try this simple test. Relax for a moment and imagine you're holding a lemon. Picture its bumpy, slightly oily skin and the bright yellow color. Now imagine taking a sharp knife and slicing into the lemon. Imagine bringing it up to your nose and sniffing that lemony scent. Now, visualize taking a bite out of one of the slices. Wait a second . . . Are you salivating? Most people do. You haven't even touched a lemon, and yet look how your body is reacting physically, just as if you had. Do you see how easy it is to manipulate your subconscious?

The lemon trick gives you an idea of how Power Programming works. The brain can't tell the difference between something you've intensely imagined, and an actual image you see before you in reality. Therefore, when you bite into that imaginary lemon, your brain triggers your salivary glands, your lips pucker, and your mouth fills with water.

When you read a book or watch a movie, your tears or laughter are quite real. In exactly the same way, the Power Programming techniques you'll learn by reading this book and listening to the CD will cause you to act in very real ways—ways that will help you master your eating and exercise habits as never before. And, of course, when you do that, you'll lose weight. Automatically.

Chuck Knoblauch, the1991 American League Rookie of the Year for baseball, illustrates just one example of the power of the subconscious. Chuck, who was playing for the Minnesota Twins at the time, was one of the most promising second basemen in the league. In 1998 he signed a four-year contract with the New York Yankees for $24 million. But after a mediocre first year with the Yankees, Knoblauch's career turned south. Suddenly, he couldn't accomplish the most fundamental task of a second baseman—throwing the ball to first base. Any Little Leaguer can do it, but Chuck Knoblauch, an all-star baseball player, couldn't. What was happening?

A few too many throwing errors caused Knoblauch to begin doubting himself, and this set a domino effect in motion. The New York media quickly picked up on Knoblauch's faltering performance and told the world about it. Then, the pressure of publicity sent Knoblauch's confidence into a tailspin, and he forgot how automatic a thing like throwing the ball to first base really was. Chuck Knoblauch had reprogrammed his subconscious to believe that he was incapable of achieving such a simple task. And that became his reality. No matter how hard he tried to force himself to succeed, he couldn't.

Chuck Knoblauch's problem is exactly the same thing that happens to people who add on pounds until they have a full-blown weight problem. Once you're overweight, you start to feel the heat. You try all sorts of fad diets and force yourself to "be good." But sooner or later, the pressure and self-doubt catches up with you and then you fail. Just like Chuck, the more you fail, the more you try to force change, and the more difficult it gets.

But here's the kicker: You don't have to force yourself to eat better. This is something you are capable of doing automatically with ease when you take advantage of the incredible power of your subconscious mind.

YOUR SUBCONSCIOUS WORKS FOR YOU AUTOMATICALLY

Have you ever struggled to remember someone's name? You think as hard as you can and the harder you try, the more difficult it is to recall. Finally, when you stop trying to remember, the name pops into your mind out of nowhere. The name comes from your subconscious, the part of your mind that makes things happen effortlessly.

When you Power Program your subconscious mind, you won't have to try hard to eat more healthfully. It will happen automatically because you'll be using the new program you've installed on your mental computer. That's exactly what happened to Daniel:

> Daniel was referred to me because he needed to lose quite a bit of weight. He knew very little about the Power Programming plan. Like many people, Daniel's eating habits were out of control. In his case it wasn't only what he ate, it was how much he ate: a huge breakfast, lunch, and dinner every day. If food was anywhere near, he ate it, whether he was hungry or not.
>
> Daniel's subconscious was overflowing with relentless cravings for food. Using Power Programming, he guided himself through a variety of imaginary scenes, such as being completely aware of his cravings at all times, but eating only when he felt hungry. This was further reinforced with images of eating healthy, satisfying foods. (During our initial consultation, we discovered which healthy foods he liked.) Tempting images of grilled chicken, peppers, and fruit filled his mind, replacing images of greasy burgers, chili dogs, French fries, and soda. Through Power Programming, he reinforced these new images in his subconscious mind.

Almost immediately, Daniel found himself eating healthful, smaller portions. And it didn't stop there! He also programmed in a new motivation to exercise. Daniel lost the 100 pounds he needed to, and best of all, he did it without a struggle. He has maintained his weight loss to this day. He learned this very important lesson: Struggle is created by the conscious mind. The subconscious mind never offers resistance. It responds to your wishes easily and effortlessly and is ripe and ready for reprogramming.

POSITIVE IMAGES LEAD TO SUCCESS

Now that you understand the basics of Power Programming, it's time to learn more about how you can use the power of images to reprogram your subconscious mind, lose weight, and keep it off permanently. The first step in achieving anything is to imagine yourself as a success, whether it's a success at work, at your marriage, or at losing weight. Here's how Jack used Power Programming to change the images in his subconscious:

Jack was 44 years old and unhappily overweight. Although he was a physician and fully understood the importance of being slim, he couldn't control himself. He snacked on ice cream every night. That's right, every night.

Jack came to me for two sessions and continued doing Power Programming on his own two to three times a week for 15 minutes at a time. Imagery was the key to his success. He imagined himself coming home from his office each night, having dinner and relaxing for the rest of the evening without any desire for ice cream. He envisioned himself going to the freezer, looking at the carton of ice cream and then closing the door with the freezer-burnt carton of ice cream still inside, and a great big smile on his face. He then imagined opening the refrigerator door and picking out a ripe piece of fruit, sinking his teeth into it, and enjoying it as if he picked it himself from a tropical fruit tree. Jack programmed these images into his subconscious mind, and he never touched ice cream again. Whenever he had one of those nighttime cravings, the first thing he thought of was fruit, and that's exactly what he reached for. By doing so, he eliminated nearly 700 late-night calories—4,900 calories a week!

If you're having trouble losing weight, you're probably fighting self-doubt and negativity in your life. Maybe you have made the decision to lose weight, but then your boss yells at you, or your boyfriend dumps you, or your spouse forgets your birthday. Before you know it, you're reaching for that carton of Rocky Road. Your failure was the result of negative, subconscious thoughts and images that led to feelings of self-doubt. This common scenario is one of the major reasons diets end in failure. But once you begin using your Power Programming techniques, belief, self-control, and confidence will surge like a raging river.

To achieve weight loss through Power Programming you need to have an open mind. Now that you have a better understanding of why Power Programming works, the process of opening your mind has already begun. You're primed and ready to succeed!

KEEP IN MIND...

Your mind is more powerful than you ever expected. Every day, you drift into altered states of consciousness, and it is during these moments that your mind becomes super-sensitive and super-receptive to change. Think about why you crave certain foods or eat such large portions. Your subconscious has been programmed to behave this way. But with Power Programming you can reprogram your subconscious with healthy, fresh images—images that will empower you to be completely in control of your eating at all times.

I'll tell you more about the remarkable power of images in Chapter 6. But right now, let's move on to Chapter 2 where you'll level the playing field and discover everything you need to know about the subconscious causes of your eating habits. The brief quiz that follows will help you understand the differences between your conscious and subconscious minds. You may be surprised at how little you know about the subconscious, your most powerful tool for change!

Which Part of Your Mental Computer Is at Work?

Decide whether each of the statements below describes the conscious mind or the subconscious mind. Circle your answer, and when you're finished, score yourself to see how well you understand the differences between the two.

1. This is the part of your mind that provides you with logic, reason, and judgment. When you eat three pieces of cake for dessert, this part of your mind will help you come up with reasons why it's okay.

   CONSCIOUS   SUBCONSCIOUS

2. This is the part of your mind that "just knows" something instinctively. When you sit down for dinner, it tells you when you've had enough to eat, even though you might not be tuned in enough to listen.

   CONSCIOUS   SUBCONSCIOUS

3. This is the part of your mind that is both aware and analytical. When you're too tired to exercise and it feels like a constant struggle to stay motivated, this part of your mind will tell you that it's okay because you put in a long day at work.

   CONSCIOUS   SUBCONSCIOUS

4. This is the part of your mind that dreams and imagines. When you can see yourself as thin and healthy, eating a delicious salad for lunch, this part of your mind is at work.

> CONSCIOUS   SUBCONSCIOUS

5. This part of your mind classifies and forms opinions about the information that is fed into it. When you beat yourself up for eating that third slice of pizza for dinner, this part of your mind is taking over, even though odds are that you'll do it again the next time.

> CONSCIOUS   SUBCONSCIOUS

6. The intelligence in this part of your mind is intellectual, not emotional. When you're feeling lonely or anxious or blue, it tells you that eating will make you feel better.

> CONSCIOUS   SUBCONSCIOUS

7. This is the part of your mind that is most receptive to helping you change your behavior. When you're doing Power Programming and you tell this part of your mind that you are motivated and in control of what you eat, it listens.

> CONSCIOUS   SUBCONSCIOUS

8. This is the part of your mind that makes excuses for poor eating habits and holds you back from losing weight. It says, "Oh, what's the use? I can't lose weight no matter what I do. I might as well just keep eating my ice cream."

> CONSCIOUS   SUBCONSCIOUS

9. This is the part of your mind that is most powerful and influences your behavior almost all of the time. When you're sitting

at Thanksgiving dinner and skip dessert because you're not hungry, this is the part of your mind that tells you to.

CONSCIOUS   SUBCONSCIOUS

10. This is the part of your mind that you work with the most during Power Programming. When you imagine yourself sinking your teeth into a juicy red apple, or jogging around a peaceful lake on a beautiful spring day, this is the part of the mind you're accessing.

CONSCIOUS   SUBCONSCIOUS

Answers

Now, check the answers below to see how well you did. Give yourself one point for each correct answer, and then add up the points to get your total score.

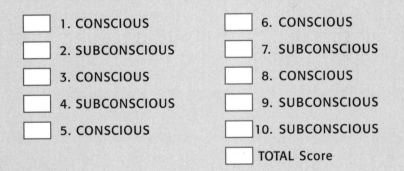

	1. CONSCIOUS		6. CONSCIOUS
	2. SUBCONSCIOUS		7. SUBCONSCIOUS
	3. CONSCIOUS		8. CONSCIOUS
	4. SUBCONSCIOUS		9. SUBCONSCIOUS
	5. CONSCIOUS		10. SUBCONSCIOUS
			TOTAL Score

CHAPTER 2

UNDERSTANDING YOUR EATING PATTERNS

You know you shouldn't have that second helping of mashed potatoes. You're fully aware of what you're doing when you reach for a bucket of fried chicken instead of a healthy salad. Even though you know perfectly well that you'll gain weight, you still clean your plate, eat when you're not hungry, and snack uncontrollably.

But do you understand *why* you cling to this self-defeating behavior? "I absolutely know that I shouldn't stop off for fast food on my way through town," Wanda says. "But I still do it. I still find myself driving up to the window and sometimes even supersizing my order."

For most people, it's not a matter of learning what foods you should or shouldn't eat. Instead, the most important first step in losing weight is to understand why you persist in your unhealthy eating habits even though you know you're working against yourself.

There are lots of environmental, social, and emotional factors that shape your eating habits. Here are the most important ones:

- *Marketing:* Marketing and advertising by food processors and restaurant chains exert a powerful influence on your eating choices. Their messages are like viruses infecting your mental computer.
- *Stress:* You may be using food to relax and ease stress. If food makes you happy, you'll reach for something to snack on every time you feel unhappy.

- *Entertainment:* Eating is a big part of socializing. Think about it. What's the focal point of almost every holiday party, vacation, or social get-together? Food!
- *Habitual snacking:* If you're like most people, you probably are in the habit of grabbing snacks that you don't really need and eating them when you're not even hungry.

THE ADS MADE ME DO IT!

The growth of the food industry has made high-fat, inexpensive meals available throughout the world. And quantity has become a major selling point. Just look at the names the fast-food chains give to their burgers. McDonald's sells the Big Mac, Wendy's offers the Big Classic, and Burger King lures you with the Whopper. What do all of these names make you think of? Size, of course. A large coke at most fast-food restaurants is as much as 32 ounces and 310 calories! When I was a kid, a large soda was about 16 ounces. In fact, just 20 years ago, kids drank an average of about 8 ounces of soda a day. Today they drink an average of 24 ounces—three times as much!

Astonishingly, a 12-ounce can of soda contains 8 to 10 teaspoons of sugar and many teens drink as many as 7 cans a day, which equals nearly 1,000 empty calories and 60 teaspoons of sugar. In fact, kids today drink twice as much soda as they do milk.

According to Eric Schlosser, author of *Fast Food Nation*, the fast-food industry makes promotional links with leading toy makers, giving away simple toys with their kids' meals and selling higher profile toys at a discount. It's a clever way to target kids. And a successful toy promotion can double or triple the weekly sales volume of children's meals. In fact, Ronald McDonald is second only to Santa Claus as the nation's most recognized fictional character. Ninety-six percent of American school children can identify Ronald McDonald before they can recognize their own name! Doesn't that tell you something?

The fast-food industry spends about 33 billion dollars a year on advertising and most of it is done subliminally, meaning that the commercials and ads affect you without your conscious awareness.

You may notice the contents of a commercial, but you probably don't realize that it's infecting your subconscious with a "virus." The purpose of advertising is to hit you where it hurts, emotionally. Recently, I watched a particular fast-food commercial showing a mom and young daughter eating burgers and fries. It seemed innocent enough, but here's what the real message was: The mother was dressed in a business suit with her briefcase, and the young girl told her mom that she appreciated spending quality time like this with her. The mom guiltily looked at her daughter while both of them smiled and ate their French fries. A working mother watching this commercial would have subconsciously absorbed the subliminal message and felt guilty without even realizing it. She would feel compelled to take her child to a fast food restaurant without consciously knowing why. Most people would agree that this kind of brainwashing exists, but in the entire history of humankind, no one who has ever been brainwashed has realized or believed it.

The food industry has done such a good job of spreading mental viruses, it's urgent for you to take defensive action. Power Programming will give you the software you need to disinfect your mental computer of insidious viruses that, if unchecked, can eventually cause it to crash.

FOOD, THE ULTIMATE PAINKILLER

Because eating makes you feel good, over time you learn to associate happiness and feeling good with food. This is one of the most compelling reasons people overeat. In fact, when you're under stress or unhappy, your mind produces hunger signals because it wants to replace stressful feelings with feelings of pleasure. In your mind, food is equated with pleasure. It acts like a painkiller, offering a quick escape from painful feelings. When a painkiller wears off, the unpleasant feelings return, and you need to take another one.

For most people, food has become a powerful remedy for emotional discomfort. When you feel stressed or unhappy, you turn to food to fill the void. If you're lonely, a bag of chips can be your best friend. If you're unhappy, a chocolate Hershey's Kiss can heal the pain. It's become second nature to most people to pair food with feelings in this way. But it isn't healthy or natural. *It's natural to eat when you feel hungry and to eat slowly and enjoy your food in moderation.* It's not natural to eat if you're not hungry, and it's not natural to quickly stuff your mouth with everything in sight.

When you experience emotional pain there's always an empty feeling inside; something is missing. Food can become the substance that numbs the pain and fills the emptiness. It temporarily relieves you from your uncomfortable feelings or circumstances. But the relief is only temporary. It doesn't solve your emotional problems. In fact, it makes them worse.

As you struggle to balance the responsibilities of life, when you find yourself coping with non-stop stress, fatigue, and worry, you may automatically reach for food to blunt the pain without even realizing it. That's what happened with Jill:

Jill was a 52-year-old woman who wanted to lose weight. During our initial consultation it was apparent that Jill's desire to lose weight was the least of her problems. Her husband, diagnosed with a rare terminal illness, was bedridden and needed 24-hour care, which she provided because she couldn't bring herself to put him in a nursing home. When she came to see me she was at the end of her rope. She was overwhelmed with stress and depression, and she had no time for herself. She was using food as a painkiller and stress-reliever, and she was eating way too much of the wrong foods, way too often. Food became her only source of comfort.

During her first Power Programming session, Jill drifted easily into a relaxed state and directed her mind toward pleasant thoughts and scenarios. She was able to accept that her husband was going to die and that she was doing everything she possibly could for him. She imagined friends and family helping out with her husband's care, giving her extra time so she could do the things she enjoyed. Power Programming provided Jill with the utmost peace, acceptance, and understanding. Her mind embraced these new images and feelings, ones she had consciously forgotten about.

The encouraging feelings she experienced through Power Programming carried over to her daily life. Not only did Jill begin eating healthfully, she began walking regularly. Jill came for three Power Programming sessions and after the final session she confessed that it had changed her life. For the first time she realized that she needed to take care of herself and that expending every ounce of her energy on her husband was unhealthy for her. Jill's subconscious mind accepted that eating was not the solution to satisfying her emotional needs. She discovered the truth through Power Programming, and now she no longer uses food to relieve her pain.

Through Power Programming, you'll be able to stop stress in its tracks. The very first thing you'll learn in your new Power Programming weight loss program will be how to develop an effective relaxation response—the one and only thing that can remove stress from your life. It's a simple technique that worked really well for Brian:

Brian was a 35-year-old stockbroker who worked on Wall Street. He had a high-pressure job, a hectic daily commute to Manhattan, and he rarely made it home before the sun went down. When he finally got home each night, he'd have about a half hour to spend with his wife and two young children. The daily grind had finally gotten to him. He missed his family, his friends, and his 32-inch waist. Brian overate as a reaction to the stress in his life and his inability to relax.

By the time I saw Brian, his blood pressure and cholesterol were sky high, and he knew he had to change, and fast! We determined that his first step would be to practice regular relaxation techniques, which are an essential component of Power Programming. Relaxation not only helped Brian to ward off stress, it also opened his mind, shedding light on the things in life that are most important, and shedding the unwanted pounds that put Brian's overall health in danger.

Through Power Programming, Brian's own mind provided the answers; he finally realized that his family and his health were more important than work. He rearranged his work schedule so that he'd be home earlier every night. He began exercising during his lunch hour, and he learned how to trigger a relaxation response whenever he became too stressed. Brian not only turned his health around, he turned his life around.

Eating to make yourself feel better is probably something you do without even realizing it. It was definitely a problem for Bonnie, a single 45-year-old woman who lived alone, worked full time, and immersed herself in snack foods every night while watching TV in an effort to blunt her loneliness:

When Bonnie came to me for help with her late-night snacking, it was obvious that snacking was causing her to gain way too much weight. The amount of calories she consumed between 8 P.M. and 11 P.M. was much more than the total calories she ate during the rest of the day. Food was her comfort, her safety blanket, and her friend. She knew she was out of control and that she urgently needed to change.

During the initial evaluation, Bonnie discussed her sewing and her Tae Bo class, a type of cardiovascular martial arts exercise, which she had been skipping regularly. The gym that offered Tae Bo was right next door to her apartment. I knew exactly what we needed to do to reboot her mental computer and switch it into weight loss mode. During her first Power Programming session, I guided her through powerful visualizations and motivational exercises. Her subconscious was programmed to believe that it would be easy to replace her snacking habits with activities that are far more comforting than eating a bag of chips or box of cookies. Also, she imagined herself doing Tae Bo during the session and this influenced her subconscious and motivated her to take action.

The following week, Bonnie came back for her next appointment with a confused, yet excited, look on her face. She couldn't understand how her behavior had changed so dramatically in just one week. She had avoided snacking completely and had gone to her Tae Bo class every night. When she was watching television she would do some sewing or ironing instead of eating. Bonnie took control of her life and became productive again, and did it easily, without struggle. She accepted herself and felt no compulsion or craving to snack.

FACING UP AND LETTING GO

Letting go of the comfort you get from emotional eating is the most difficult obstacle to overcome. Food becomes your safety blanket; it becomes your medicine for relieving stress, depression, or tension. But when you look in the mirror and see the pounds piling on, you feel even worse. It's difficult to let go of the safety blanket, but if you don't, you'll be setting yourself up for more serious emotional issues later, not to mention serious weight problems.

"Why me? Why do I do this to myself? Why do I allow myself to get so heavy?" These are questions you ask yourself when you continue to eat for emotional reasons. Eventually, you muster up the strength to go on a diet, but diets don't eliminate the reasons for overeating, and eventually you return to the old destructive patterns. You'll continue to have weight problems until you address the emotional attachments you have to food and discover the positive feelings hidden deep inside of you. Your Power Programming techniques will allow you to download those positive feelings, just like they did for Madeline:

Madeline was 100 pounds overweight and desperate. She worked full time, was raising a young child, and suffered from depression. Another therapist who didn't specialize in weight loss referred her to me. The other therapist told me that Madeline was terrified of giving up food. Madeline's husband left her a year earlier. She was not close to her siblings or parents and had been constantly made fun of as a child. During our first consultation, Madeline confessed that food was the only thing she had left to hold on to.

Initially, when we started the sessions, Madeline was subconsciously resistant. Her fear of change was so intense that it prevented her from letting go and opening her mind, so I focused the sessions on a technique called regression. It involves self-acceptance, motivation, and self-control to help break down these resistances.

All of your past experiences are stored away subconsciously. When debilitating emotions linger, as they did in Madeline's case, it means that the feelings haave never been dealt with, accepted, and released. Regression is a technique in which you mentally revisit the scene that initially triggered the negative emotions. Eventually, Madeline was able to identify and accept the cause of her negative feelings, and let them go. She uncovered the motivation, self-control, and discipline that she'd locked away inside. These new feelings were enough for Madeline to finally detach herself from emotional eating. She no longer relied on food to feel good. She lost the 100 pounds she needed to lose, and not surprisingly, her depression subsided.

When you feel depressed, anxious, or stressed, these uncomfortable emotions become so overwhelming that the good, positive feelings we all have buried inside seem nonexistent. Switching from negative to positive is a habit that takes practice, but it can be done and it will enhance your ability to lose weight using Power Programming.

Losing weight doesn't have to be difficult. You probably know exactly what eating habits led you to gain weight, but it helps to understand why they exist and where they came from. This understanding will make your mind more receptive to the power of suggestion, a key component in Power Programming that you will learn about in Chapter 6.

FOOD AND FUN

We eat and drink to celebrate holidays, birthdays, anniversaries, graduations, weddings, and promotions. Getting together with friends usually means meeting at a restaurant or spending time at home eating a meal or having snacks. One thing's for sure, no matter where the gathering takes place, there had better be some good food!

I was recently invited to a friend's house for a get-together and I took careful mental notes about the role of food at the event. As expected, the moment my wife and I arrived we were offered a drink and I noticed a variety of appetizers readily available for everyone to enjoy. In our society, this is expected. In fact, it would be considered socially unacceptable to invite guests over and *not* offer anything to eat or drink. Unfortunately, this evening didn't seem like much fun for the hosts; for them, it was work, work, and more work. And what all of the work entailed? You guessed it: preparing and serving food.

It started with potato chips, nachos, and dips—and then the appetizers were rolled out while everyone stood around talking and sipping cocktails. Pigs in a blanket, shrimp cocktail, bruschetta, and mushroom pastries circulated throughout the room. From a corner, I tracked how much food one of my friends ate during the evening: nine pigs in a blanket, four shrimp, two bruschettas, and six mushroom pastries, not to mention the chips and dip.

Eventually the "real food" was served, buffet style. There was penne a la vodka, chicken marsala, roast beef, potatoes, and several other items (too many for me to remember). I wondered how anyone could actually be hungry at this point. This party confirmed for me a common trend we can all identify within our culture: The focal point of friendly get-togethers is always food.

It's important for you to be aware of this overemphasis on food and how much you actually eat when you're socializing. I know that my friend (the one who gobbled up all those appetizers) had no idea how much he was eating, how many calories he consumed, or *why* he was even eating. The social distractions prevented him from noticing how much he ate. In effect, he was on automatic pilot because he was at a party where everyone was expected to eat. His mental computer was programmed this way. Furthermore, when dinner was announced, he didn't hesitate to fill up on more food. Could he possibly have been hungry at that point? Absolutely not! Then why did he and just about everybody else continue to eat? Because their subconscious minds were conditioned to associate food with pleasure.

On average, each guest at the party consumed between 2,000 and 3,000 calories, far beyond the recommended daily calorie intake of 1,800. And this was just one meal! No wonder 65 percent of Americans are overweight! Carol's story is a typical example of how Power Programming can help you avoid all of those unnecessary calories in social situations:

> When Carol came to see me, her eating was completely out of control. If food was around, she ate it. She ate so much that even she couldn't believe it. When she returned for her second visit, I asked her how she did between sessions. "I guess I did OK," she said. She told me that she'd gone to a wedding the previous Saturday. When I asked her how she handled herself with the eating, she hesitated; she hadn't realized what she'd done until I asked. During the cocktail hour, she had one beer and two hors d'oeuvres. "That's strange," she said. "Normally I would have had twenty hors d'oeuvres and five beers." I asked her if she was exaggerating and she said "absolutely not." Her mind was so receptive to all we did during the first session that she didn't even notice how it had influenced her choices! It became mindless. In the past, the cocktail hour would have been a race against the clock for Carol. She'd have been eating and drinking as quickly as possible so she wouldn't "miss out" on anything.

For her, programming her subconscious to eat only when she was hungry made weight loss a reality. And, most importantly, it felt normal to her. In fact, her new response became so natural and automatic that she hadn't even noticed how well she'd been doing. It had already become second nature.

John, a 37-year-old client of mine who loved to combine food with travel, is another example of how Power Programming can help you control your eating in situations that are designed to influence you to overeat.

John eventually came to me to help him control his eating, which had really gotten out of control on his last cruise. I saw John for three sessions, and he did quite well. John was surprised at how his new eating habits had become so automatic. When we were getting ready to schedule his fourth appointment, he told me that he'd be going on vacation to Club Med the following week and was afraid that he'd lose control of his eating. His biggest fear was the "greeting room" that guests enter upon arrival, which would be overflowing with a smorgasbord of food. This was Club Med's way of welcoming its guests. Little did he know, this concern was actually his saving grace. In the past, John would have dived right in the moment he walked through the greeting room door, but now, his concern meant that he was aware of the triggers and the risks. And awareness is the first sign of improvement.

During his Power Programming sessions, I guided John through the entire scenario. He imagined walking into the greeting room with his head held high, feeling confident and in control. He directed his attention to the other people in the room and how they were eating. This made him feel free and realize how ridiculous uncontrolled eating really is. The session put John in touch with his ability to control his ingrained habits, something he hadn't felt in a long time.

When he returned from his trip, John told me that he did, indeed, enter the greeting room feeling super-confident. Right away, he noticed how everyone else in the room was shoving goodies into their mouths as fast as they could. Then a feeling of peace swept over him, and he felt driven to eat light, healthy foods. Discipline and self-control became normal for him, and greatly outweighed any urge to eat uncontrollably. His mind accepted these new responses without a problem, and he was completely immune to the temptation to join in when others around him were gorging themselves on food.

SNACKING, GRAZING, PICKING, AND BINGING

Endless snacking has always been considered a no-no, but many people feel helpless when the kitchen cabinets are bursting with cakes, chips, and cookies. It's as if there's a magnetic force drawing them to the very foods they should be avoiding. Does that sound like you? If so, you probably fall into one or more of these categories. Are you. . .

- a subconscious snacker and picker?
- controlled by your cravings?
- a lunchtime salad eater?
- a weekend or nighttime binger?
- a dishwasher?

A Snacker and Picker

Whether you're munching on goodies throughout the day or diving into a bag of chips during your favorite TV sitcom, you probably pick on food between meals even though you've told yourself many times before that you're going to stop. Most of the time when you're snacking, you're not even hungry. You're locked into the habit of snacking throughout the day or during specific activities. The next time you have the urge for a snack, ask yourself, "Am I really hungry?"

Claire was a typical snacker and picker:

When we sat down for the first time to discuss Power Programming and weight loss, Claire confessed that she did pick and snack, but she didn't realize how much this affected her. It didn't seem like a big deal to her because she would eat little bits and pieces at a time. What she didn't realize was that the bits and pieces added up. She would grab handfuls of M&Ms in the office, and pieces of cake or cookies if they were around. At home she'd eat cookies and ice cream most nights, when she wasn't even hungry. In fact, after we analyzed her typical day, we concluded that her snacking was adding approximately 500 extra calories a day to her diet.

The key with Claire was awareness. She wasn't hungry when she munched on candies or gobbled down cookies. She did it because of habit and temptation—insidious viruses that infected her mental computer. During her Power Programming sessions, I suggested to her subconscious that she would eat only when hungry and at no other time, and that anytime she was about to eat something she would become instantly aware of her hunger. These suggestions were combined with imaginary scenes at work and at home. She imagined walking into a co-worker's office, seeing a great big bowl of M&Ms, immediately noticing that she wasn't hungry, and easily avoiding them. She imagined sitting on her porch after dinner, recognizing her non-hungry feeling and being perfectly content, with no need to grab cookies or ice cream.

Claire Power Programmed her mind to pay attention to her hunger signals, not her cravings and habits. Her mind had accepted that she would eat only when hungry and that doing so would be easy, not a struggle. Her picking and snacking habits vanished, the viruses in her mental computer disappeared, and so did 20 pounds of excess weight!

For many people, if food is there, they eat it. That was the problem for Mary, a 55-year-old mom who needed to lose 30 pounds:

> Mary ate a healthy, sensible breakfast and lunch each day, and cooked dinner almost every night. In fact, cooking was Mary's passion. But when she cooked, she subconsciously picked on the food she was preparing. When dinner was ready, she wasn't hungry, but she ate the whole meal anyway. Not only was she taking in lots of additional calories, she was doing it at night when her body's metabolism was at its slowest.
>
> Through Power Programming techniques, Mary became aware of what she was doing. Without any effort, she stopped picking, and she also unearthed an intense motivation and discipline to exercise and cook healthier meals. Her subconscious welcomed these new, healthy behaviors while eliminating the old fattening ones. The last time I spoke with her, Mary was 35 pounds lighter. Not only did she achieve her goal, she surpassed it!

Controlled By Your Cravings

Some people have cravings so powerful and so deeply rooted in the subconscious, they can't fight them on a conscious level. Betty was one of those people:

> When Betty arrived at my office, she was desperate for help. For someone who considered herself poised, organized, and motivated there was one monkey on her back that she couldn't shake. Every time she drove past a Burger King or McDonald's, she couldn't resist pulling in and binging on the burgers and fries. At times, she'd force herself to keep on driving, only to end up turning around farther down the road. Betty explained to me that these cravings were so unbearable when she drove past these places, she felt as if she morphed into another person. The very sight and smell of a McDon-

ald's or Burger King were enough to trigger images of tasty golden fries and juicy flame-broiled burgers. She knew how unhealthy it was and she knew she wasn't even hungry when it happened. It had nothing to do with hunger; it was the marketing, advertising, and branding of fast food that had her brainwashed.

By using Power Programming, Betty trained her mind to erase these cravings and compulsions from her mental computer. During her sessions, she imagined herself driving past fast-food places, smelling the aroma in the air, seeing the large signs and feeling disgusted by all of it, not tempted. Instead, she created an image of discipline and control, without any cravings at all. Between sessions, Betty purposefully drove past fast food joints without even slowing down, and loving every minute of it—something she never thought she'd be able to do. She used her mind to free herself from her prison, and lost 25 pounds, permanently.

A Lunchtime Salad Eater

Another game many people play is limiting themselves to "just salad" for lunch. I've worked with dozens of overweight people who eat very light breakfasts and lunches, maybe just a salad and a glass of water, yet they're not able to lose weight! How can this be? Salad is healthy, as long as it's not smothered in Thousand Island dressing, but by itself it's not enough to give your body the energy it needs to get you through the day. You end up feeling famished by late afternoon, and you wind up overeating later on in the evening. If you "do the salad thing," probably you want to believe that you're making a concerted effort to lose weight, and you love the attention and admiration you get from your workplace lunch buddies for being so good. Then, when you don't lose weight, you tell yourself that you've tried your best, and nothing will ever work—a perfect excuse for falling back into our old eating habits. That's what happened with a former client of mine, Rich, who thought he had it all figured out:

All Rich needed to do to lose weight was have a bowl of cereal in the morning and salad for lunch, and he'd lose that 50 pounds, or so he thought. When he finally decided to make an appointment with me, he was at his wit's end; after four weeks, the salad thing wasn't working. When I interviewed him, I asked him about his other meals. I knew the breakfast and lunch situation, but I didn't know what happened after that. His response was that he ate pretty much whatever he wanted for dinner because he ate so healthfully throughout the day. But that was the problem. The amount of food he ate at dinner and the speed at which he ate it was out of control. Furthermore, he did a lot of late-night snacking. What it boiled down to was this: Because Rich was taking in so few calories during the course of the day, he became famished by dinnertime. Rich was actually taking in more calories at night than he had been before he started his new salad diet. Here's how Power Programming helped.

Rich drifted into a deep, relaxed state of mind in no time, making his subconscious super-receptive. I asked him to imagine enjoying his cereal for breakfast and feeling in control. I threw in a suggestion that at 10:30 A.M. he would feel the need for a snack, like a yogurt or banana. As the session progressed, we got to lunch. Rich imagined eating salad, but with tuna or grilled chicken mixed in. He also imagined eating fruit and a slice of bread if he was still hungry. Next I threw in a suggestion that in the afternoon, when he was feeling hungry, he would eat a granola bar and a piece of fruit. Then I had him imagine feeling slightly hungry instead of starved when dinner approached. He imagined eating slowly, feeling in control and consuming much less, and doing it easily and without effort.

Rich's mind accepted all of these images and suggestions, and he found it easy to control his behaviors. He lost the 50 pounds he needed to lose along with the feelings of intense hunger.

Thousands of you salad eaters out there have a deep, dark secret that your coworkers don't see! When evening rolls around, that cool, in-control salad eater that everyone admires disappears! If you're a lunchtime salad eater, you might get by with as little as 400 calories during daytime hours. But when dinnertime rolls around, you may consume as many as 2,000 calories in just 15 or 20 minutes, followed by more binging throughout the night. Then you go to bed with a full stomach when your body's metabolism is at its most sluggish, and the pounds start piling on. In fact, between 11 P.M. and 11 A.M., the body's digestive ability drops to 18 percent of its normal daytime effectiveness. Your body stores this late-night calorie overload instead of burning off that extra energy, which is the most certain way to gain weight.

Your mind is also part of the problem here. Because you do well all day long with your small breakfast and sensible lunch, you probably feel justified in eating pretty much whatever you want at night. But, ultimately, if you eat like a bird all day, you're starving your body, leaving it no other option but to store nighttime calories as fat. By severely limiting your intake during the day, you're also depriving your body of important nutrients, such as protein. This can lead to a drop in blood sugar, which triggers a craving for foods high in starches and sugars.

To break this cycle, you need a healthier, more balanced eating plan. A turkey or peanut butter sandwich and a piece of fruit will provide your body with the protein and fiber it needs. Healthy snacks to nibble on, such as a protein bar or handful of air-popped popcorn, will help to ease the intense evening hunger, cravings, and binges. Then you don't have to worry about your mind playing tricks on you. Check out the healthy eating tips in Chapter 4 for suggestions on how to enhance your Power Programming weight loss plan with healthy foods that will keep you satisfied, and thin!

A Weekend Binger

Just because you earn high marks for good eating behavior Monday through Friday, it doesn't automatically follow that you'll win the battle of the bulge. Steve is proof of the fact that calories don't respect the days of the week:

> Steve was 300 pounds the first time he arrived at my office. He was 42 years old, single, and worked hard. He ate very healthfully and immersed himself in exercise all week, but when Friday evening arrived he turned into a walking time bomb. He usually found himself at the local bar where he would binge the entire weekend on alcohol and food. He told me that he could open his refrigerator a hundred times Monday through Friday and have absolutely no desire for the icy bottle of Grey Goose Vodka on the shelf. But when he got to that bar everything changed; he couldn't control himself. Steve's subconscious had formed a connection between the bar and "going all out."
>
> During his sessions with me, Steve imagined himself in the controlled state he was in Monday through Friday, and he really enjoyed the feelings of self-control and confidence. I asked him to build upon these feelings during his sessions and imagine them growing and expanding. Then I asked him to imagine walking into the bar with all of these feelings fully expanded. He imagined having just a couple of drinks, eating normal-sized portions, and feeling in control. I suggested to his subconscious that he would be in control 7 days a week from now on. I reinforced this suggestion several times.
>
> When Steve came back for his next session, he told me that for the first time he was able to go to the bar and control himself. He said it felt empowering and encouraging. He continued this pattern no matter where he was, and he got his weight down to 180 pounds. In a very short time, Steve was able to reprogram his mental computer with software that guided him to eat and drink sensibly, and to be in control of his unhealthy eating habits.

Weekend binging is certainly a problem that can stem from an overly controlled daytime diet. Monday through Friday you eat like a champ, you exercise with great dedication, and you seem to have everything under control. Then the weekend rolls around, you have a couple of days off, and you let loose. You treat yourself by going out for a couple of cocktails followed by a big dinner and maybe a gooey dessert. Saturday morning comes and it seems okay to have bacon and eggs instead of your usual banana and yogurt or whole-grain cereal. Perhaps you treat yourself to another big meal on Saturday night. After all, it's the weekend! You've worked hard all week.

But when you eat like this, you'll always have a hard time losing weight because you sabotage those good weekday eating habits, and eventually slip up completely. You then wonder why you can't lose weight. You think you're doing everything right, but eventually you give up completely and begin eating destructively again, not just on the weekends, but all the time.

Of course, it's okay to go out for a nice meal, but when you do this to reward yourself for good behavior, there's a tendency to go overboard. It's certainly possible to go out for a nice meal and enjoy it without overeating. When you Power Program your subconscious, you won't *want* to order the biggest, unhealthiest entrée on the menu. The important thing is to find the right balance so that eating healthfully is easy and struggle-free. And it all begins in the mind.

A Dishwasher

Many people feel the need to clean their plate when they eat, even if they're not hungry anymore. If this sounds like you, it's not that you can't control your behavior. It's that you haven't learned *how* to control it, at least, not yet. That was the problem for my client Bobby:

> Bobby was a 40-year-old bond trader who ate a sensible breakfast and lunch each day, but his downfall was dinner. At 7 P.M. every night, he would sit down at the dinner table and gulp down everything on his plate, even if the portions were huge. And it had nothing to do with his level of hunger. He would almost finish his entire meal before his wife could even

put a dent in her meal. And he never left food on his plate. Bobby was out of control. He felt disgusted going to bed every night stuffed and bloated. No matter how hard he tried, he couldn't stop these dinner binges that were causing him to gain a lot of weight.

Using Power Programming techniques, Bobby learned how to visualize himself eating in a controlled, deliberate fashion. He created a mental picture of himself sitting down at the dinner table, eating in slow motion. When he did this, his mind had enough time to tell his stomach he'd had enough.

Before discovering Power Programming, Bobby's subconscious was programmed to wolf down his food and clean his plate. He learned as a young kid that it was wrong to waste food. After his Power Programming sessions, he ate slowly, ate less, and savored every bite. He felt satisfied, not full, and the new non-full feeling allowed him to lose 30 pounds in three months. But it didn't end with this! Bobby also found himself seeking out healthier foods and exercising regularly. He no longer felt guilty for throwing food out. He was finally in complete control, and he loved it.

What is it that makes people like Bobby eat so much? One reason is that we're taught at a very young age that it's wrong to throw away food because of all the people starving in the world. Another reason is portion size; we've become accustomed to super-sizing our food and when we try to do otherwise, it feels like we're not eating enough. Our subconscious gets sucked into these habits. But it's vitally important to remember, no matter how much food is on your plate, you should eat only when you're hungry. And you should keep portion sizes on the small side. It takes much less food to satisfy your hunger than you think. Supersize your portions, and you'll supersize your waistline!

KEEP IN MIND...

Before you can use Power Programming to its full potential, it's important for you to understand your subconscious eating patterns. This chapter has shed light on the environmental, social, and emotional factors that lead to overeating. When you tackle these factors head-on by reprogramming your mental computer, you'll discover the secret to painless and permanent weight loss. Whether you're an emotional eater, a snacker, a binger, or a hostage to your food cravings, you can Power Program your subconscious mind to change your fundamental eating habits and achieve permanent weight loss without pain or effort.

Let's move on to the next chapter, which will explain the reasons behind a critical truth you already know: In the long run, diets just don't work! But first, try out the quiz that follows and measure your awareness of your eating habits and the calories you consume each day.

Raising Your Eating Awareness

Awareness of why you eat, when you eat, and where you eat is essential in developing a healthier eating lifestyle and preparing yourself for Power Programming. If you're like most people, you don't think about how many calories you consume in a day and you don't know why you eat the way you do. When you identify and confront the things you need to change, you prepare your subconscious mind for Power Programming that will make the change happen.

To take the quiz, circle the answer that best describes you for each of the questions below:

1. How long did it take you to eat your last meal?

   a. 10–15 minutes
   b. 15–20 minutes
   c. 20–30 minutes

2. How many servings of food did you have at your last meal?

   a. 1 serving
   b. 2 servings
   c. 3 servings

3. At what point during your last dinner did your hunger first disappear?

   a. In the beginning
   b. Somewhere in the middle of the meal
   c. When I felt full

4. How much food was left on your plate when you were done with your dinner?

   a. None
   b. Very little
   c. A good amount

5. How did you feel when you finished eating?

   a. Very full
   b. Moderately full
   c. Satisfied but not full

6. How much food did you eat at your last meal?

   a. A lot of food
   b. Not enough food
   c. Just the right amount of food

7. Describe the calories in most of your meals?

   a. High in calories
   b. An average amount of calories
   c. Low in calories

8. How many healthy snacks do you consume on average every day? (fruits, vegetables, granola bars, yogurt)

   a. 0 servings
   b. 1–2 servings
   c. 3–4 servings

9. How many unhealthy snacks do you consume on an average day? (cakes, cookies, chips, candy)

   a. 0 servings
   b. 1 serving
   c. 2 or more servings

10. What were the total calories of yesterday's snacks?

    a. 100–200 calories
    b. 200–300 calories
    c. Have no idea

11. When you eat salty snacks such as potato chips, approximately how many do you have?

    a. 10–20 chips (or other salty snack)
    b. 20–30 chips (or other salty snack)
    c. 30 or more chips (or other salty snack)

12. How did you feel the last time you snacked?

    a. Very hungry
    b. Moderately hungry
    c. Not hungry

13. How often do you pass-up free treats, for example, cake left in the office?

    a. Always
    b. Sometimes

c. Rarely

14. How many sweetened drinks (soda, iced tea, juices) do you consume in an average day?

a. None
b. 1–2
c. 3–4

15. How many sweetened drinks did you consume today?

a. None
b. 1–2
c. 2–4

How High Is Your Eating Awareness?

For each question, read the explanation below and circle the number of points you earned. Then, add up all of your earned points to get your total score. The explanations below will help you interpret your total score and find out how high your eating awareness is:

80–90 points	Excellent! Your eating awareness is very high.
60–80 points	Very Good. You're on the right track.
40–60 points	Not bad! You're almost there.
40 points or less	Not to worry! Change is just around the corner.

1. If you chose (C), you are eating at a good pace. Many people tend to eat fast, which usually translates to overeating. Once you begin your Power Programming sessions, your awareness will be sky high, and you'll never race through meals again.

A = 2 points   **B = 4 points**   **C = 6 points**

2. The best answer is (A), but be careful. Food labels can be mislead-
   ing. Often, portion sizes are much larger than they need to be. Eat
   the amount of food you need to get rid of your hunger feeling, and
   not one bite more.

   A = 6 points   **B = 4 points**   **C = 2 points**

3. (B) is the best answer here. You want to make sure that you eat
   slowly so that somewhere in the middle of your meal you're beginning to feel satisfied.

   A = 4 points   **B = 6 points**   **C = 2 points**

4. (C) is the best answer. Work on leaving a good amount of food on
   your plate. If you chose (B), that's a good start. If you chose (A),
   you'll be on track soon enough.

   A = 2 points   **B = 4 points**   **C = 6 points**

5. The safest way to eat is to stop when your hunger goes away, which
   is quite different from stopping when you feel full. So (C) is the best
   answer. As you use your Power Programming exercises, you'll begin
   to realize that you never want to feel full again.

   A = 2 points   **B = 4 points**   **C = 6 points**

6. The best answer is (C). You always want to eat just the right amount
   of food. Eating too little could set you up for a crash. Eating too
   much could mean that you're consuming too many calories.

   A = 2 points   **B = 4 points**   **C = 6 points**

7. (B) is the best answer. You want to consume just the right amount
   of calories. As you progress with Power Programming, you'll discover
   yourself becoming much more in tune with your body and you'll
   develop an awareness of how much is just right.

   A = 2 points   **B = 6 points**   **C = 4 points**

8. If you chose (C), great. You should eat 3-4 servings of healthy snacks per day. If you eat 1 or 2 (B), that's good. If you don't typically eat something light between meals, you'll start to.

   A = 2 points   B = 4 points   C = 6 points

9. Obviously (A) is the best answer, but a sweet treat every so often is not going to kill you. As you move through Power Programming, you won't even want to eat unhealthy snacks.

   A = 6 points   B = 4 points   C = 2 points

10. Tough question here. If you selected (A) or (B), that's good. It's important to know how many calories there are in the snacks you eat. But if you chose (C), not to worry. Power Programming will give you the awareness lift you need.

   A = 6 points   B = 6 points   C = 2 points

11. Another awareness question here. It's not too often that we know how many chips we've had. If you selected (A), then you're already on the right track. Good job.

   A = 6 points   B = 4 points   C = 2 points

12. (B) is the best answer. It is best to eat a light snack as soon as you feel a twinge of hunger. That way you don't starve yourself and wind-up overeating later.

   A = 4 points   B = 6 points   C = 2 points

13. Although (B) isn't bad, (A) is better; it means you are in total control. If you selected (C), don't panic. That's about to change.

   A = 6 points   B = 4 points   C = 2 points

14. If you selected (A), hooray! Three cheers! What a relief! The average 12 ounce soft drink contains 8 teaspoons of sugar and 140 calo-

ries. If you do drink soda, after doing Power Programming you won't even want it anymore.

A = 6 points   **B = 4 points**   **C = 2 points**

15. Again, (A) is the best answer.

A = 6 points   **B = 4 points**   **C = 2 points**

CHAPTER 3

WHY DIETS DON'T WORK

Every day, millions of people fight carbohydrates, fat, and calories, and every day they're getting fatter and fatter. What's going on? It's certainly not because there aren't plenty of diets to try! Dieting is a 40 billion dollar-a-year industry, yet more people are overweight now than at any time in history.

According to the National Institutes of Health, 95 percent of diets fail. That doesn't mean people don't lose weight on these diets. They do. But while millions of dieters lose weight, only five percent keep the weight off. Those who do keep the weight off are successful not because they changed their diet, but because they actually changed their lifestyle. And lifestyle change can only come from the mind.

PLAIN AND SIMPLE, DIETS DON'T WORK. HERE'S WHY:

- Diets depend on willpower. While you might have strong willpower at the beginning of a diet, over time, the subconscious cravings that control your eating habits are much stronger, and they win out in the end.

- All diets focus on food, and you can't ignore what you're trying to avoid. In fact, your mind will draw your attention to the very foods you want to avoid, and trigger powerful cravings.

- Diets try to make you change your comfort zone, which is extremely difficult to do, unless you change the thinking of your subconscious mind.

SUBCONSCIOUS CRAVINGS VS. WILLPOWER

Most dieters spend a lot of time counting points, calories or carbs while ignoring their most powerful resource: the mind. Your cravings for food come directly from your subconscious mind, so it makes sense that the only way to change these habits is to access the subconscious. Yet diet programs try to help you lose weight through conscious, rational methods. Trying to rationalize your way through food cravings is about as helpful as holding your breath when you're having an asthma attack. It just doesn't work because it's not targeting the source of the problem. That's where Power Programming comes in. It works to eliminate food cravings embedded in your subconscious mind. That's why it works every time and it lasts forever.

The idea behind every diet plan is simple: Eat fewer calories. No matter how fancy the diet, each one typically outlines a plan for you to do what you already know you need to do—change the way you eat. You think these regimented plans are the ticket to controlling your eating habits, but they don't work that way because they don't really change your habits.

When you start a new diet, you "will" yourself to stick to the program. You hang on for as long as you can, but eventually you slip and fall. Those cravings and compulsions programmed into your subconscious are like an itch that's just too insistent. Sooner or later, you have to scratch. Inevitably, you slip off the diet, cheat a few more times, then a few more, and soon you've gained back the weight. A few months later, you're ready to try the next fad diet. The term for this is *yo-yoing* and for Stephanie, it was a predictable cycle that had been going on for years:

> Stephanie was a professional "yo-yoer." She holds the record in my book for losing the most weight over the years. She also holds the record for gaining back the most weight. Stephanie tried every diet imaginable, lost weight every time, but never kept it off. She explained to me that dieting made

her miserable. The whole time she was dieting, all she thought about was food, and her cravings triumphed every time. She could follow all the diet plans in the world, but it didn't matter; none of them eradicated her cravings for food.

Stephanie came back to the office a week after her first session of Power Programming and she told me that she felt as if she'd escaped a 10-ton weight. She was no longer burdened with thoughts of food. She began to eat sensible portions, never thought about snacks, had no desire for desserts, and eventually lost 80 pounds! Her food cravings disappeared completely. Most importantly, she lost her title for gaining back the most weight!

It was quite simple for Stephanie to rid her mind of nagging food thoughts. All along she had been trying to consciously push these thoughts out of her mind. It didn't work, because the thoughts were programmed into her subconscious through years of reinforcement. Power Programming allowed Stephanie to go directly to her subconscious, and rewrite the program. Once she reprogrammed her subconscious with images and suggestions of self-control, sensible eating, and eating healthier foods, everything clicked into place. She got to the source of her problem and was able to change her eating habits permanently.

DO YOU YO-YO THROUGH LIFE?

Here's how yo-yoing begins for most folks. It's January 1 and you're ready to lose 10 pounds on the latest miracle diet, eating nothing but cabbage, lettuce, and low-fat frozen meals every day. This will lower your calorie consumption to 1,100 a day, 700 calories less than the recommended 1,800 for losing weight. You also join a gym so you can burn off another 300 calories, shrinking your calorie total to 800 a day. That means you're taking in 1,000 less calories than the recommended 1,800, and you should therefore lose one pound every 3½ days, or two pounds a week.

You feel great and stick to your diet program for five weeks, and lose the 10 pounds. But something else happens. You become famished and riddled with cravings. All you can think about is gobbling up a Big Mac and an entire box of Ho-Hos. Before long, you just can't take it anymore, and the next thing you know, you careen off your diet. At this point, you probably go on a giant binge, and then go right back to your old eating habits. All of the weight you lost creeps back along with a few additional pounds. Before you know it, you're back in the red zone.

Two months later you start all over again on a new diet.

You see, cravings are so powerful and so firmly programmed into your subconscious mind that they'll always sabotage your conscious mind's willpower. Dieting alone hasn't worked for you in the past because when you diet you force yourself at a *conscious* level to change your eating habits. The only way you can actually change your eating habits is to go directly to the source of your cravings: your *subconscious* mind.

I'm sure you've met many yo-yo dieters in your life. You may well be one of them. But after you use Power Programming to lose weight, your yo-yoing days will finally be over!

ARE YOU A FOOD FANATIC?

When you diet, what are you thinking about morning, noon, and night? The carrots and celery you can eat. The bag of lettuce you can mix with tuna. Food. Food. Food. . . *The worst thing about all diet plans is that they focus on food.*

"When I'm not dieting," says Kara, a 52-year-old professional, "I don't think about food that much. But as soon as I go on a diet, that's *all* I think about. What am I going to make for lunch? How big will my portions be? What foods can I have?"

As Kara discovered, your attention is drawn to exactly what you're trying to avoid in the first place: food! Your mind automatically thinks about food first and foremost, and that creates intense cravings. For example, take the Weight Watchers program. It uses a point system to help you keep track of the food you've eaten. Every time you record your points, you have to think about the foods you've eaten that day. Moreover, it will make you think about the bad foods you couldn't eat, and that will trigger your cravings.

In time, your frustrated compulsions and pent-up desire for food will accumulate until they snowball out of control. Let me put it to you this way: *Diets make you think about being hungry.* Remember, your subconscious mind is programmed to eat large portions, supersize your meals, and reward yourself with cake, cookies, and chocolate. And dieting can't possibly change these mental programs. Change takes place on the subconscious level only. Any diet can help you lose weight initially, but rarely does any diet help you keep the weight off permanently. The more stringent the diet is, the harder it will be to maintain the weight loss after you go off the diet.

The Atkins Diet is another popular diet that, like Weight Watchers, may work at first. But it doesn't achieve permanent weight loss. The Atkins diet takes an unorthodox approach: avoid carbohydrates, eat foods that are high in fat and cholesterol, and bingo, you lose weight! Although loading up on protein-rich foods and avoiding carbs sounds like the master plan for reducing fat and building muscle, when you fill up on protein-rich foods such as meat and dairy products and cut out carbs, you miss out on essential vitamins. Avoiding carbs lowers blood glucose levels, causing the body to crave sugar for energy. This almost always leads to junk food binges. Furthermore, a lack of carbs depletes muscle-glycogen levels, forcing the body to convert muscle tissue into glucose for energy.

People on low-carb diets often lose weight rapidly, but the kind of eating that's required can't be maintained for a lifetime. Furthermore, medical experts warn that loading up on bacon and steaks can lead to long-term health risks such as heart disease, stroke, kidney problems, and ulcers. Nevertheless, you put on your blinders and insist, "I can have all the hamburgers and steaks I want as long as I avoid breads and fruits." That's like saying, "I can pump my arteries full of cholesterol and put myself at risk for heart disease as long as I lose weight."

Atkins and other low-carb diets have created a national obsession about avoiding bagels, breads, and pastas, which has created a neurosis about carbohydrates, and an even stronger desire to eat them. You can't walk into a supermarket or restaurant these days without coming across a low-carb section. Gabriella was an innocent victim of this low-carb craze:

> When Gabriella arrived at my office, the first thing she said to me was that she needed to avoid carbohydrates because she was addicted to them. This wasn't the first time I heard this from a client. When did carbohydrates suddenly become an addictive substance? I wondered, "Should they be made illegal?"
>
> I explained to Gabriella, as I do with all of my "carb-crazed" clients, that she'd been persuaded through media, supermarket shelves, restaurant menus, and gossip to believe carbs are the cause of the overweight epidemic in our country. Sure, Gabriella enjoyed pasta and good Italian bread, but so do the Italians, and most of them aren't overweight! Eating an occasional bowl of pasta didn't make her heavy. She was overweight because she ate too much and didn't exercise enough. Carbohydrates became her justification for being overweight, her alibi. The real problem was that she just liked to eat, and wasn't ready to admit that she needed to change her lifestyle. Actually, she was afraid to change.
>
> After some brief counseling about the real source of her weight problem, she began her Power Programming sessions. The first session focused on breaking down her faulty perceptions about carbohydrates and accepting that she'd still enjoy eating, but consume less of the food on her plate.
>
> Next, I transmitted powerful images and suggestions for a new eating style to her subconscious mind. She imagined eating in a controlled, disciplined fashion, learning to pay close attention to her "hunger feeling." She discovered during her sessions that it felt much better to stop eating when the

"hunger feeling" went away, not when she felt full. After that, every time she sat down for a meal, she automatically honed in on her hunger feeling and sought out that "just right" feeling.

When she returned for her next session, she was amazed at how in-control she felt. She was no longer crazed about carbohydrates or afraid of having to give up eating. After some careful calculations, we estimated that she had reduced her dinnertime calorie intake alone by nearly 400 calories. She lost 20 pounds in less than two months, and still enjoyed her breads and pastas, just in lesser quantities. And she did it without any struggle at all!

CHANGING YOUR WAYS

Eating less and exercising more is the only real formula for losing weight. Pretty simple, right? Interestingly, this formula doesn't seem so simple to anyone who is trapped in their habits and ways. Changing your ways is like climbing Mount Everest. It's awfully challenging, but every so often you try it anyway. You drum up the motivation to diet and probably have some success, but sooner or later you inevitably revert back to your old ways. Your "ways" are nothing more than your mindset—your thoughts put into actions. They are how you define yourself.

Whenever you try to change the way you do things, whether it's eating in a controlled manner or exercising regularly, you are forced out of your comfort zone. Sure, you want to change the way you look and you want to improve your health, but deep down inside, you just don't like to change the way you do things. Instead, you say to yourself, "I think I'll try out this new diet. It looks easy, and I don't have to sacrifice too much. I'll only have to make minor changes." Although you know you should exercise, you can't get yourself to do it because exercising seems about as exciting as having a root canal.

This is pure perception! Once you use your mind to hyper-link fun, achievement, motivation, and success to exercise, it will become something that you *want* to do. Power Programming will help you program in the link and change your perception. I've worked with hundreds of people who once hated to exercise, and I've watched them become passionate about it as a result of Power Programming. When achievement and reward are connected to exercising, it can become your passion, too. The same rule applies to changing your eating habits. Just ask Donna:

> Donna was a 59-year-old retiree and grandmother of four who came to see me about Power Programming for weight loss. I discussed with her the importance of regular physical activity in losing weight. She chuckled, "I'm not the exercising type." You hear these kinds of expressions all the time. "I'm not the dancing type," or "Cooking isn't my thing," or "The outdoors is just not me." Donna needed to step out of her comfort zone, change her habits, and change the way she perceived herself if she really wanted to lose weight.
>
> During her Power Programming sessions, she saw herself trying new things. She imagined herself going out for a daily walk with her neighbor Betty, enjoying the fresh outdoors and friendly companionship. After all, Donna considered herself to be a very social person. This imagery was further strengthened with power suggestions like these:
>
> - Because you are a social person, you enjoy a brisk, social walk with your friend.
> - Exercising is something you now do and enjoy.
> - You can be anything you want to be.
> - You can do anything you want to do.
> - Only you can tell yourself what you are or what you aren't.
>
> After a couple of sessions, Donna felt different about herself. She started realizing that she was tired of being the same old Donna. "Who says I'm not the exercising type?" she demanded. She realized that the most successful people in the world are those who challenge themselves and take risks. She

unpeeled the labels she had attached to herself, freed herself from her preconceived notions, and lost the 35 pounds she wanted to lose.

Remember, your "ways" are the thought processes that determine your actions. Trying to change your actions without changing your thoughts won't work. Once you become a master of Power Programming, you'll break free from your past and develop new life-long habits. You'll lose weight and keep it off without a struggle.

CRAVING HEALTHY FOODS

What about that five percent of people who actually keep the weight off after dieting? Why are they successful while the other 95 percent aren't? The answer is simple: after those dieters lost weight, they kept it off by making a life-long commitment to healthy eating and exercise. The ones who gained weight back never made a commitment to anything. Their weight loss was driven entirely by willpower. And willpower is never more than a temporary fix.

Any goal or commitment begins with a thought, and the stronger the thought, the better the chance of success. Here's an example of how powerful your mind is and how quickly it creates involuntary actions:

Take a moment to think about your favorite food. Now close your eyes and imagine yourself eating that food. Try to vividly feel the texture as you chew and allow your taste buds to experience the rich, vibrant flavors. Now open your eyes and see if you've salivated.

What kind of food were you imagining? I bet you were thinking about a food that isn't very healthy. (If you *were* thinking about something healthy, like a juicy piece of pineapple, congratulations! You're already on the right track!)

Close your eyes again. This time, imagine eating your favorite fruit. Feel your teeth sink into its soft body as the cool juices tickle your taste buds. Feel the juices slide smoothly down your throat and into your anxious stomach.

Did you salivate again? If you thought about unhealthy food the first time you did this exercise, it's because your subconscious mind is littered with images of these foods. But you salivated while thinking of the healthy food, too! This is because you like these foods, even though your subconscious doesn't realize it yet. When you start to practice Power Programming methods, you'll automatically begin to crave healthier foods.

Using Power Programming to lose weight isn't limited to restructuring your thoughts about food; it also helps facilitate self-control, discipline, and motivation. When these characteristics are combined with your healthy food thoughts, weight loss and weight maintenance not only become real, they become easy.

The next time you see someone who has lost weight and maintained it, ask how they did it. I'll bet the person tells you it was easy! That's because the person has committed herself mentally to staying slim. She's integrated healthy images and thoughts into her psyche and convinced her subconscious—although she may not know it—that eating less, eating healthier foods, and exercising is okay. These people have learned to harness healthy thought processes. They aren't dieters; they're realists.

Like juggling or riding a bike, losing weight is three-quarters psychological. Once you learn how to juggle, you never forget it, just like you'll never forget how to ride a bike even if you haven't been near one in 30 years. Even playing the piano comes back to you, no matter how long it's been since you practiced. Once your mind learns something, it's always there. Once you have figured out how to tap into your subconscious to lose weight, it will permanently become a part of you. You will lose weight and keep it off—effortlessly.

KEEP IN MIND...

You can't will yourself to avoid cravings. If you try, you'll end up with the 95 percent of dieters who fail. Willpower functions on a conscious level, while eating and exercise habits are driven from a subconscious level. The only way you can overcome your food cravings is to reprogram your subconscious, something that dieting doesn't do. Instead, dieting very often deprives you of the nutrients you need. A healthier, more permanent method of weight loss involves three things: (1) making sensible food choices from all food groups, (2) eating frequently and regularly in moderation, and (3) exercising. Power Programming will make it natural and effortless for you to achieve success in all three.

Before you move on to Chapter 4, where you'll discover healthy eating tips to enhance your Power Programming techniques, try the Dieting Diary that follows and see how much insight you can gain into your own personal weight loss struggle.

Your Dieting Diary

Answer the following questions and see for yourself if dieting works. Thinking about your answers will help you sort out some of your feelings about losing weight. Remember, if you haven't succeeded at losing weight and keeping it off, it's not because you failed. It's because the diet failed. I'll repeat what I've already said many times: diets just don't work for permanent weight loss.

After you've answered the questions, read the analysis that follows and see if you recognize yourself!

1. Name all the diets you can think of that you have ever tried.

_____

_____

_____

_____

_____

_____

_____

2. How many of these diets actually worked for you and for how long?

_____

3. If you found success with any of your diets, why aren't you on that diet now?

_____

_____

4. How many times have you lost weight on a diet, but then gained the weight back?

_____

5. What do you think were the reasons that you gained the weight back?

_____

_____

6. Was dieting ever easy for you?

_____

7. Did you ever crave food when you dieted?

_____

8. What's the longest amount of time you were able to maintain your weight loss when dieting?

_____

9. What was the reason for maintaining weight loss while on a diet?

_____

10. Do you think you will ever diet again?

_____

Do You Recognize Yourself?

1. Name all the diets you can think of that you've ever tried.

   Most likely, you've been on many different diets, and you've probably forgotten to include a few here. But the important point is that your chances of failure with any diet are 95 percent. You have only a 5 percent chance of success. The problem is not with you. It's with the method. Diets simply don't work.

2. How many of these diets actually worked?

   Well, you're reading this book, aren't you? That means that the diets you've tried so far have not worked. Weight loss results from a lifestyle change that lasts a lifetime. If you've gained back weight that you lost with a diet, then the diet didn't work.

3. If you found success with any of your diets, why aren't you on that diet now?

   Diets teach deprivation, making them impossible to stay on.

4. How many times have you lost weight on a diet, but then gained the weight back?

   If you've gone on a diet, gained the weight back, and then gone on another diet, you are a yo-yo dieter. At best, yo-yo dieting doesn't work. At worst, it can damage your health. Power Programming can cure you of the yo-yo diet syndrome.

5. What were the reasons for gaining the weight back?

   Binge eating is the body's natural response to excessive dieting. The more you diet, the more you think about food, and the more you feel the need to eat. Eating regularly and in moderation is the best defense against binge eating.

6. Was dieting ever easy for you? How did it make you feel?

You probably answered no to this question. Dieting can lead to irritability, withdrawal, depression, and intense cravings. As you learned in this chapter, it just doesn't work.

7. Did you ever crave food when you dieted?

You almost certainly have answered yes to this question. Most diets lead to a preoccupation with food and it is even common to experience dreams about food.

8. What's the longest amount of time you were able to maintain your weight loss when dieting?

Remember, anyone can lose weight, but very few people can keep it off. And keeping it off is what matters. Maintaining your weight is a life-long commitment and it can only be achieved if you change your subconscious thoughts about food and eating.

9. What was the reason you were able to maintain a healthy weight while dieting, even if it wasn't permanent?

This is sort of a trick question. What you should really be thinking is "What was the reason I stopped maintaining my weight." Losing weight through dieting can create a rush similar to gambling. You might have some success initially and think you've got it all under control, but then you go broke. You crash, because dieting involves willpower and willpower is only temporary. The odds are always against you.

10. Will you ever diet again?

Even if you answered yes to this question, you'll be very happy to learn that you won't need to diet ever again after you Power Program your subconscious mind.

HEALTHY EATING TIPS TO ENHANCE POWER PROGRAMMING

I know you're anxious to begin your first Power Programming session, BUT WAIT! The following pages provide important guidelines and tips to help you shape good eating habits by clearly defining your eating goals.

The guidelines I'm about to give you will help you focus on healthy eating habits before you even begin your first Power Programming session! Whether you're a late-night snacker, an overeater, or something in-between, Power Programming will be more effective if you define and organize your goals, thoughts, and strategies in your mind before you attempt to reprogram and reorganize your mental computer. The following guidelines are designed to help you do just that. Along the way, I'll give you some weight loss secrets I've discovered in many years of working with people just like you.

TIPS FOR LATE-NIGHT SNACKERS

Eating a few healthy snacks during the day helps you keep your energy level steady by spreading the calories you consume throughout the day so that you don't feel the need to overeat at meals. Endless snacking at night, after dinner, *isn't* good, and it's not something your body needs. Most people snack at night because they're bored, or because it's just part of their habitual routine. Downing a bag of chips or a bowl of ice cream at night while you watch your favorite TV program is one of the worst ways to snack and one of the best ways to gain lots of unwanted weight.

The goal of Power Programming is to train your subconscious so that you'll control snacking instead of letting snacking control you. It may not be possible to eliminate late-night snacking altogether, but you'll certainly be able to train your mind to snack only on healthy foods. Here are some steps you can take right now to prepare your subconscious for the changes that are about to take place:

1 **Buy healthier snack foods.** Potato chips, cookies, and Ring-Dings don't magically appear in your cupboard. The only reason they're there is because you decided to buy them. Although your Power Programming sessions will weaken your cravings for junk foods, start preparing your subconscious by removing these foods from your house right now. If junk food isn't there when the cravings strike, you won't eat it.

2 **When you want a snack late at night, eat something that's healthy.** Start filling your fruit basket with some of your favorite fruits. Stock up on those juicy treats now. This will further empower your subconscious to prefer fruit over junk food when you begin your Power Programming sessions.

3 **If you feel a tweak of hunger at 9:30 P.M., think small.** Most late-night snackers gain weight because they eat too much when they snack. Now's the time for you to start thinking small. If you let yourself, you can go through half a bag of potato chips or half a box of cookies in the blink of an eye. So, if you absolutely must have cookies, limit it to two small ones, and resist the urge to have the whole box. Remember: Start thinking small now. You can also experiment with the dozens of brands of low-fat and low-sugar cookies available today. You'll find one that you like, and you'll save calories even on two cookies. Power Programming will help you reinforce this habit easily.

4 **Drink a cup of warm decaffeinated tea.** Herbal tea can be very calming and keep you busy so that you steer away from boredom eating. Chamomile tea, made from whole organic chamomile flowers, promotes relaxation and is especially useful before bed. Other popular teas that have health benefits are orange spice, ginseng root, and ginger lemon.

5 **Prepare healthy snacks ahead of time.** If you have a pineapple sitting on your counter, cut it up and put it in the fridge. A lot of late-night snacking choices have to do with convenience. It's a lot easier to tear into a bag of Doritos than to slice up a messy pineapple when you're sitting on your couch watching the evening news. If the pineapple is all cut up and ready to go, you're much more likely to eat it. Or, mix a large container of plain yogurt and granola, and divide it into small portions to stash in the fridge for those late-night cravings. (They also make a great breakfast treat!)

TIPS FOR SUPER-SIZERS!

Most people have a tendency to underestimate the amount of food they eat. Within the last 20 years, portion sizes have ballooned out of control and it's gotten to the point where nobody knows what a normal-sized portion is anymore. Maybe you eat larger portions than you need because you finish everything on our plate, even when you're not hungry anymore. Maybe you eat huge portions because you wait until you're famished, and then you eat way too fast and way too much!

How portion sizes have changed

When you look at how much portion sizes have changed over time, it's not hard to see why today one person in five is obese:

- In the 1980s a typical bagel was three inches in diameter and about 150 calories; today it's ballooned to six inches in diameter and 350 calories, more than twice as much.
- In the 1980s the average cheeseburger was a little over 300 calories; today's average cheeseburger is a little less than 600 calories—almost double the size.
- A large cup of soda topped out at 16 ounces in the 1980s. Today the max is 64 ounces. That's one half gallon!—four times as much.

- In the 1980s the average serving of French fries was 2 ounces and 210 calories. Today's average-size portion has tripled to more than 6 ounces and 600 calories.
- A typical turkey sandwich just two decades ago yielded about 350 calories; today it tips the scale at more than 800 calories— a 228 percent increase.
- In the 1980s, an average muffin was 1½ ounces and 210 calories; today it's 5 ounces and 500 calories. Yikes!
- One slice of cheesecake was 250 calories in the 1980s. Today it's more than 600 calories, big enough for two or three people!
- A chocolate chip cookie 20 years ago was about 1½ inches in diameter and 55 calories; today's large cookies are nearly 300 calories each—a 545 percent increase. A colossal difference!

What portion sizes should look like

With a little practice, you can estimate the calories you're about to eat just by looking at the quantity of food on your plate. Here are some guidelines that will tell you what adequate portions should look like.

- A serving size of vegetables or fruit should be the size of a fist.
- A serving of meat, fish, or chicken should be the size of a deck of cards.
- A cup of ice cream should be the size of a billiard ball.
- A serving of nuts should be the size of a ping-pong ball.
- A serving of cheese should be the size of a business card.
- A baked potato should be the size of a computer mouse.

You Don't Have to Clean Your Plate!

No matter how much food is piled on your plate, you eat all of it, right? If that's what you do, you're not alone. You probably learned about the clean plate club when you were a child and your well-meaning parents told you not to waste food because there are starving children elsewhere in the world. But don't worry; Power Programming will help you develop enough self-control and independence to take care of this problem. For now, here are some quick tips to help get you started:

1 **Become aware that you're finishing everything on your plate out of habit, not hunger.** This is the first step. When you're tuned in to your behaviors, they become easier to change. Once you begin using Power Programming, you will hone in on the plate of food in front of you and want to eat sensibly.

2 **Eat slowly and enjoy every bite.** When you focus on every bite and eat slowly, you enjoy your food more. Feel the texture on your tongue and enjoy the flavors of every bite. This will give your mind enough time to tell your stomach that you've had enough.

3 **Understand that throwing away food isn't wasting it.** The idea that you're wasting food if you don't eat all of it is one of the biggest contributors to the obesity epidemic in our culture. Think about it. Isn't being gluttonous also being wasteful?

4 **Never keep eating until you're full.** Your body wasn't meant to feel full. There is a big difference between eating until you're satisfied and eating until you're full. When you feel full, it means that you have grossly overeaten.

Eat Slowly!

Many people practically wipe their plate clean before others at the table have even had a taste. If you're one of them, it's probably because you wait until you are famished before you allow yourself to eat. This is one of the most common reasons that people overeat. Here are some tips to avoid overeating due to extreme hunger:

1 **Become aware of how fast you eat.** Your Power Programming techniques will condition your subconscious to do this, but

you can start to get the ball rolling right now, and it will enhance the receptiveness of your subconscious when you begin your Power Programming sessions. This may sound a little strange, but try it anyway. Put a small spoon in your pocket and carry it with you at all times. You'll notice it throughout the day and it will serve as a continuous reminder to eat slowly.

2 **Eat small, healthy snacks throughout the day.** Most people who are speed eaters are so hungry when their meal is in front of them that they just can't wait. Make sure that you aren't completely famished before any of your meals. Try a banana in the middle of the afternoon when you need a boost. Another good trick is to eat half of your sandwich for lunch and save the other half for later. This is an excellent way to spread out the calories and avoid that starved feeling.

3 **Drink a lot of water.** Water can work wonders for curbing your appetite. Make sure you sip water all day long so that you consume about six to eight glasses a day.

4 **Eat a lot of fiber.** Fiber makes you feel fuller longer because it stays in your stomach for a while, slowing down your rate of digestion. If you're between meals and you start to feel a little bit hungry, have a snack full of fiber so that you don't feel starved later on. Try some apple slices with a little peanut butter, or be a little daring and give roasted soybeans a try; they're loaded with fiber and much tastier than you may think. If these snacks aren't appealing, how does a fruit smoothie or yogurt sprinkled with granola sound?

TIPS FOR WORKPLACE EATING

The workplace can be a haven for weight gain. You spend lots of time at work and your body naturally becomes hungry during these hours. When you're surrounded by vending machines loaded with candy and soda, lunch trucks filled with hot dogs and chips, and meetings accompanied by donuts, cookies, and Danish, it can be easy to forget to plan ahead. Here are some quick tips to help you start developing new habits right away:

1 Store the following foods at your workplace:
   - Bottled water
   - Canned fruit
   - Cereal
   - Cottage cheese
   - Dried fruit
   - Fresh fruit
   - Granola bars
   - Rice cakes
   - Salads
   - Skim milk or soy milk
   - Vegetables
   - Yogurt

2 When you have to eat at a meeting
   - Eat a granola bar or a piece of fruit right before your meeting.
   - Drink a bottle of water before the meeting. Water helps curb your appetite.
   - If your meeting is early in the morning, have breakfast first. This way you won't rely on donuts and Danish for breakfast.
   - Sit on the opposite side of the room from the food.

3 When vending machines are your only option
   - Buy bottled water instead of soda.
   - Eat pretzels instead of potato chips.
   - Have a granola bar instead of a chocolate bar.
   - Go a different route so that you don't have to pass the vending machine.

TIPS FOR BOREDOM EATING

Nearly half of all adults turn to food to conceal feelings of boredom or loneliness and it usually happens subconsciously. You don't even think about it as you absentmindedly munch on food. But don't worry. Power Programming will awaken your motivation and awareness to help you stop the mindless munching. In the meantime, here are some of the things you can begin doing now to kick-start your motivation and awareness:

1   **Double-check your hunger.** Most of the time when you eat out of boredom, it has nothing to do with hunger. Even if you think you're hungry, double-check to make sure you're really hungry and not just bored or lonely. Awareness is the key to avoiding eating for the wrong reasons.

2   **Drink a glass of water.** Before you reach for food, drink a glass of water and wait 10 minutes. Sometimes thirst can seem like hunger.

3   **Do something active.** Sometimes you're not remotely hungry, but just looking for something to do. Get up and do a load of laundry, go for a walk, or call a friend. This will take your mind off boredom and food.

TIPS FOR MAKING BETTER FOOD CHOICES

Now, let's really start getting your mind prepared for Power Programming. Certainly you know that eating healthy foods is an essential part of weight loss, yet you can't help but eat the unhealthy, high-calorie stuff. You might even be in denial about the amount of calories those foods contain. In fact, I bet you have no idea how many calories there are in most of your food choices. Here are a few of the most common problems we all have when it comes to food choices, and helpful solutions for each one. Recognizing these problems and identifying solutions will enhance the vividness of the images you program into your subconscious during your Power Programming sessions:

BREAKFAST

Common Challenge: Although it's tempting, a ham and cheese omelet is not the best way to start your day. It has 490 calories, 38 grams of fat, and 716 milligrams of cholesterol. It may taste delicious at first, but you'll pay a heavy price later, and there are other foods that will satisfy you just as much, if not more.

Power Solution: Most omelets contain three eggs. A good way to cut some calories and cholesterol is to ask for your omelet with one regular egg and two egg whites. Or you can get an all-white omelet. Instead of ham and cheese, load-up your omelet with fresh vegetables like mushrooms, tomatoes, onions, or broccoli. You'll enjoy your omelet and it will actually be good for you! If you have to have cheese or meat, try fat-free turkey sausage or fat-free or low-fat cheese. You won't know the difference!

· ·

Common Challenge: Do you have the urge to eat McDonald's hot-cakes and sausage? Many of us do. But how do 770 calories and 33 grams of fat sound? How about the McDonald's deluxe breakfast? Do 1,220 calories and 60 grams of fat float your boat? Although these fast-food breakfasts can be tempting, they spell disaster for your health and your weight.

Power Solution: If you like to eat a quick breakfast out, keep it simple. A McDonald's English muffin with grape jam or strawberry preserves is just 185 calories and 2 grams of fat. Or you can go to your favorite diner or coffee shop, sit at the counter, and order that egg white omelet I suggested earlier. Tell your server that you have to get to work, and you'll be out of there in no time. You can always prepare your own breakfast at home and stay away from take-out breakfasts entirely. Try some apple cinnamon oatmeal before you leave your house. It's simple to make and contains just 180 calories and 2 grams of fat.

· ·

Common Challenge: Are breakfast sandwiches your thing? Think again! Bacon, egg, and cheese on a bagel can add up to 500 calories and 29 grams of fat. Want one of those pints of chocolate milk to go with it? Then tack on an additional 460 calories and 16 grams of fat. The calories add up more quickly than you think, and a drink like chocolate milk can add lots of unnecessary calories to your meal.

Power Solution: If you want to have a breakfast sandwich, try a low-fat bagel with a little bit of light or fat-free cream cheese instead. You can have a glass of fat-free chocolate milk, too, without tipping the scales! Or do your body a favor and try some low fat yogurt with sliced strawberries. It's only 200 calories and it's a great energy-booster for the morning.

Common Challenge: Think most muffins are healthy? They may be the comfort food you think you need in the morning, but today's bakery muffins can contain as many as 630 calories, without butter or any other spreads. That's not very comforting!

Power Solution: Try a low-fat or fat-free muffin, but be careful of the size. A whole-bran muffin with raisins is a good choice, but make sure it's not too big. They're much healthier for you and they contain loads of fiber.

Common Challenge: Many of us are fans of those big country breakfasts. But get this: Two fried eggs, buttered toast, and four strips of bacon can set you back 500 calories. That's a lot of calories for just one meal—especially your very first meal of the day!

Power Solution: If you must have eggs, ask for them poached; it's a lot healthier than fried eggs. Put a little jelly on your toast instead of butter, and ask for a side of fruit instead of bacon. If you really want a healthy breakfast, go for the whole-grain cereal with 2% milk and a sliced banana. It's only around 200 calories, very refreshing, filling, and very healthy.

....

LUNCH & DINNER

Common Challenge: Most of us crave a McDonald's Big Mac, large fries, and a large coke sometimes. But the value meal contains 1,410 calories and 92 grams of fat. Throw in an apple pie for dessert, as delicious as it may seem, and you've just added 250 more calories and 11 more grams of fat, bringing your total to 1,780 calories and 66 grams of fat.

Power Solution: Go for the McDonald's Caesar salad with grilled chicken. It has just 210 calories and 6 grams of fat. For dessert, try the fruit 'n yogurt parfait; it's just 130 calories and 2 grams of fat and delicious!

....

Common Challenge: If you get a craving for two chili dogs with cheese, think about the fat you'll be putting into your body unnecessarily. This quick meal is about 850 calories and a staggering 54 grams of fat.

Power Solution: For an equally delicious and satisfying hot dog meal, try fat-free or low-fat hot dogs. Two of them with mustard and sauerkraut add up to a mere 330 calories and 3 grams of fat and you won't taste the difference. Enjoy!

....

Common Challenge: Pizza is an all-time favorite lunch or dinner for almost everyone, especially parents who are looking for a quick dinner before soccer, dance lessons, or hours of homework. But the typical pizza meal consists of three slices of cheese pizza and a can of soda. This quick meal will quickly add a whopping 730 calories to your waistline!

Power Solution: Instead of eating three slices, which you don't need to satisfy your hunger, have one slice and a side salad. Or try pizza without the cheese, or pizza with vegetables. There are lots of delicious alternatives to try until you find a new favorite!

· ·

Common Challenge: Those chicken parmigiana or meatball heroes everybody loves can spell disaster for your weight. They can be anywhere from 600 to 1,000 calories and up to 50 grams of fat—way too much for one meal!

Power Solution: Order the grilled chicken sandwich with lettuce and tomato and add a little honey mustard. That's just 320 calories and 12 grams of fat. Your body will thank you, and so will your stomach!

· ·

Common Challenge: An Italian hoagie (sub) contains ham, salami, cheese, and oil piled high on a 6- or 10-inch roll. It's a heart attack waiting to happen. Can you guess how many calories you'll consume with just one hoagie? Try 1,400 calories and 90 grams of fat on for size! It's just not worth it!

Power Solution: A turkey breast sandwich will yield just 215 calories and it's delicious and very satisfying. You'll feel good and look good after a meal like this!

· ·

THE POWER PROGRAMMING FOOD PLAN: HEALTHY CHOICES MADE EASY

The Power Programming food plan is all about making balanced and healthy eating choices. I've put together a couple of aids to help get you pointed in the right direction, even before you begin with your first Power Programming session. By thinking on a conscious level about the right food choices, you'll prime your subconscious mind for reprogramming that will end your dieting days forever!

In the pages that follow, you'll find Quick Guides that will help you stock up on the right kinds of foods. You can photocopy the

Quick Guides and take them with you to the supermarket to make shopping easier.

I've also provided sample menus for a full three weeks of delicious, balanced meals prepared with fresh, whole foods instead of the high-calorie, low-nutrition processed foods that line supermarket shelves. You can follow the menus exactly, or use them as a guideline to help you design your own balanced, nutrition-packed meal plans.

The important things to remember are:

- Eat healthy, whole foods
- Eat modest portions
- Eat slowly
- Eat only until you feel satisfied

Bon appétit!

Quick Guide BREAKFAST

EAT HEARTY	STAY AWAY FROM...
Whole grain cereal with skim or 2% milk	Sugar cereals
Sliced banana	Pancakes with butter & syrup
Yogurt	Bacon
One half whole-bran muffin	Blueberry muffins (including low fat)
Oatmeal	Hashbrowns
Fruit salad	Egg sandwiches
Unsweetened orange juice	Sweetened juices
Farina	Bagel with butter / cream cheese
Whole grain toast (no butter)	Conventional omelets
	Breakfast sausage
	Biscuits & gravy

Quick Guide LUNCH

Eat hearty	Stay away from...
Turkey sandwich without mayonnaise	Mayonnaise
Grilled chicken wrap with vegetables	Hot dogs
Grilled chicken club	Hamburgers
Fish	French fries
Vegetable wrap with vinegar	Cheese steaks
Salad with grilled chicken	Soda
Salad with salmon or tuna	Fried chicken
	Tacos
	Pizza
	Egg salad
	Penne with vodka sauce

Quick Guide DINNER

Eat hearty	Stay away from...
Plenty of vegetables	Steak that is not lean
Chicken	Pizza
Fish	Burgers
Brown rice	Hot dogs
Salads	Baby back ribs
Broccoli	French fries
Asparagus	Tater Tots
Spinach & greens	Cheeses
Tomatoes	Butter
Eggplant	Tacos
Sweet potatoes	

WEEK 1

Power Programming Menu

	BREAKFAST	LUNCH	DINNER
MONDAY	Raisin Bran with skim milk	Turkey sandwich with lettuce, tomato, and mustard	Penne sautéed in garlic and olive oil, with mushrooms and sun-dried tomatoes
TUESDAY	Cheerios with skim milk and sliced bananas	Tuna sandwich prepared with light mayonnaise, topped with lettuce and tomato	4-ounce salmon fillet with pesto sauce, accompanied with steamed broccoli
WEDNESDAY	Apple and cinnamon oatmeal prepared with 2% milk	Grilled chicken wrap with vegetables, light Monterey jack cheese, and cilantro	Grilled quesadilla with avocado and scallion
THURSDAY	Whole-bran muffin with a glass of orange juice	Grilled chicken salad with walnuts and vinaigrette dressing	Vegetable pizza without cheese
FRIDAY	Egg white omelet with onions and peppers	Turkey sub sandwich	Rigatoni with sautéed onions and fresh cherry tomatoes
SATURDAY	Life cereal with skim or soy milk	Light vanilla yogurt mixed with oatmeal and a side of fruit salad	Turkey burger served with spinach salad
SUNDAY	Fruit salad and yogurt	Chicken tacos in a corn tortilla, topped with low-fat cheddar cheese, shredded lettuce, and diced tomatoes	Broiled lemon chicken with capers served with a side of asparagus

WEEK 2

Power Programming Menu

	BREAKFAST	LUNCH	DINNER
MONDAY	Wheaties with skim milk and sliced strawberries	Turkey breast on rye with a slice of cheese, lettuce, tomato	4-ounce lean sirloin steak with a sweet potato
TUESDAY	Assorted fresh fruit and a half of an English muffin with jelly	Sushi	Grilled shrimp kabobs
WEDNESDAY	Fresh granola with skim milk and grapefruit juice	Salmon burger with light Dijon mustard	Boneless pork chops with peas and carrots
THURSDAY	Whole bran muffin with juice	Turkey sub sandwich	Chicken and vegetable stir-fry over rice
FRIDAY	Egg white omelet with tomatoes and peppers	Grilled chicken on a roll with balsamic vinegar, lettuce, and tomato	Lemon zest sole or flounder with a side of vegetables
SATURDAY	Multi-grain cereal with skim or soy milk	Vegetable wrap with portabella mushroom	Rotisserie chicken and vegetables
SUNDAY	Egg white and tomato on a honey-wheat English muffin	Sushi	Grilled chicken and vegetable kabobs

WEEK 3

Power Programming Menu

	BREAKFAST	LUNCH	DINNER
MONDAY	Organic cereal with skim milk	Yogurt parfait with unsweetened granola	Tacos with organic, all-white meat chicken
TUESDAY	Oatmeal with a glass of orange juice	Grilled chicken strips over mixed greens with mango salsa	Whole wheat pasta dressed with chopped, sautéed onions and peas
WEDNESDAY	Organic cereal topped with blueberries and sliced strawberries.	Smoked turkey breast with honey mustard on whole grain bread	Breaded chicken breast, lightly sautéed and then baked, topped with arugala & diced tomatoes
THURSDAY	Whole bran muffin with juice	Turkey wrap with avocado and shredded spinach	Chicken and vegetable stir-fry over brown rice
FRIDAY	Whole grain toast with smooth peanut butter	Steamed, peeled shrimp with tropical fruit salad	Grilled swordfish with asparagus and sweet potato
SATURDAY	Multi-grain cereal with skim or soy milk	Spinach salad with grilled chicken, raw mushrooms and sliced strawberries	Rotisserie chicken and vegetables
SUNDAY	Strawberry smoothie with slice of toasted whole grain bread	Ham and cheese sandwich (lean meat) with light Swiss cheese and mustard on rye bread	Salmon (prepared with chili garlic rub) sandwich on whole grain bread with lettuce and tomato and a side salad

PART TWO

Relaxation, Imagery,

and Motivation:

The Keys to

Power Programming

RELAXATION: THE LINK TO YOUR SUBCONSCIOUS

Relaxation is the first and most important step in Power Programming your mind to lose weight permanently. Relaxation unlocks the door to your subconscious mind, so it is absolutely essential for you to be in a state of deep relaxation in order for Power Programming to work. Think of relaxation as the password that gives you access to your mental computer. Without the password, you're locked out of the computer. But when you have the password (when you are truly relaxed) you can go into your mental computer (your subconscious) and install new software for losing weight quickly and easily. Your subconscious mind will run the new software, your eating and exercise habits will change, and excess pounds will melt away.

But before going further, it's important for you to understand that the kind of relaxation I'm talking about is something quite different from the kind of relaxation you might be accustomed to. Lying down in front of the TV with a bag of chips in one hand and the remote control in the other *isn't* true relaxation. Nor is guzzling down a couple of cocktails in a crowded, noisy bar. *True* relaxation doesn't numb the mind, it nourishes it.

When your body and mind are physically relaxed, your metabolism, heart rate, and blood pressure all drop automatically. Your subconscious mind opens, and your thoughts become quieter, sharper, and more focused. True relaxation enables you to access your mental computer so you can reprogram it however you wish. Once you achieve true relaxation, you trigger what I call your body's natural *relaxation response*. When the natural relaxation response switches on, your stress response switches off, making it impossible for you to be stressed. As I stated earlier in this book, you cannot be both relaxed and stressed at the same time.

In a moment I'll outline a series of brief warm-up exercises that will help you achieve a state of general relaxation and will demonstrate for you what it means to trigger a relaxation response. These exercises, which take less than five minutes to do, will lower your heart rate, breathing, and blood pressure and will noticeably reduce mental and physical tension. Here's how a simple relaxation exercise enabled Ken to overcome his worry and stress:

> Ken was a 28-year-old English teacher who put a lot of pressure on himself. He spent a lot of time worrying about grading papers and dealing with the department administration. Ken came to see me because he had gained 40 pounds over the past two years, and he knew that he was eating way too much. He found his eating habits "impossible" to control. During Ken's initial consultation, it became evident that he was engaging in stress eating. He constantly worried about work, which led him to seek comfort in food. The first thing we needed to do was reduce his stress.
>
> During Ken's first Power Programming session, he was restless at first, but eventually he drifted into a deep, comfortable, relaxed state of mind. I suggested to him that the relaxed feeling he was experiencing could be attained at any time. I told him that all he needed to do was take three deep breaths and say to himself, "calm and relaxed." This suggestion stuck with Ken like glue. Whenever he started to think about stressful work and deadlines, he would catch himself, take three deep breaths and repeat to himself, "calm and relaxed." That phrase became the hot button Ken could push at any time to trigger a relaxation response. After practicing this for one week, Ken told me he felt much calmer and better. He also noticed that he was eating a lot less, and he realized that he no longer needed food to relieve his stress.

In two more Power Programming sessions in my office, Ken continued to acquire tools for alleviating stress and increasing control over his eating habits. He also continued to use his "calm and relaxed" tool. In the end, Ken was able to recognize stress approaching and to head it off using various relaxation tools and techniques. In 8 months he lost the 40 pounds he had gained and felt better than he had in years. Not only was he much thinner, he was calm and stress-free all the time, and he was able once again to find enjoyment and pleasure in his life.

If you, like Ken, eat as a means of dealing with stress, you will actually be making your stress worse and setting yourself up for more serious health problems in the future. When you learn to trigger a relaxation response, you'll not only put an end to stress, you'll also unlock the door to your subconscious mind where you can use Power Programming to change your eating and exercising habits.

The ability to trigger a relaxation response starts with the simple act of breathing.

PROPER BREATHING: THE FIRST STEP TO RELAXATION

Before I show you some simple warm-up relaxation exercises, you first have to learn how to breathe properly. Although breathing supplies your body with oxygen, its most basic need, amazingly very few people know how to breathe properly. By learning to improve your breathing you will not only induce a deeper relaxation response, you'll also enhance the overall effectiveness of your Power Programming sessions.

When your breathing is shallow, it deprives your brain of the oxygen it needs to function at its best. Insufficient oxygen consumption weakens bodily functions and prevents blood nutrients from doing their job. It also slows down circulation, causing you to have cold feet and hands, fatigue, and fuzzy thinking. Technically, a person who's barely breathing is barely alive. By contrast, a pattern of deep, slow breathing carries oxygen through your blood and nourishes all the cells in your body.

Here are some basic breathing techniques you can begin practicing right away to achieve a relaxation response. Practice these breathing techniques regularly, until you can consciously use them in place of your old, shallow breathing habits. The better you are at it, the more effective Power Programming will be for you. Choose any one of the following breathing exercises, or you can mix and match. They are all equally effective. Each of these exercises will take about five minutes to complete. You should find a quiet, comfortable place to sit, recline, or lie down, such as a couch, an easy chair, a recliner, or a carpeted floor. Practice these techniques once a day for about a week.

Belly Breathing

1 Find a quiet and comfortable place to recline or lie down. It's best to lie flat on your back with your knees slightly bent.

2 Place your hands on your abdomen and take deep, slow breaths, feeling the movement of your abdomen as you breathe. At this point, while you're still breathing, begin to focus on specific parts of your body that you're relaxing and nourishing with oxygen.

3 Close your eyes and imagine a dark, comforting color.

4 As you imagine the color, inhale slowly, counting to 5.

5 Hold the breath for 3 seconds.

6 Exhale for 6 seconds, making sure that all of the air in your lungs has been exhaled completely.

7 Repeat the exercise, slowly breathing in and exhaling 25 times. As you breathe slowly and deeply, imagine that your blood is cleansing and healing all of the cells of your body.

8 As you continue practicing this technique, gradually increase the count until the inhalation rate is 10 seconds and the exhalation rate is 15 seconds.

Interval Breathing

1 Breathe in and out slowly and deeply several times to relax your body.

2 Count to 7 while you inhale, and count to 10 as you slowly exhale.

3 Inhale again, but this time inhale for 9 seconds and exhale for 12 seconds.

4 Repeat this technique two more times until your inhalations and exhalations last for the entire count. The more you practice and the more slowly you breathe in and out, filling and emptying your lungs, the more deep breathing will feel natural to you. That will help facilitate the deeper level of relaxation that is used during Power Programming.

Nostril Exchange Breathing

This is a common yoga exercise. Just as you have a dominant hand, you also have a dominant nostril. Some people are left-nostril breathers and others are right-nostril breathers. Practicing this technique will help you create more consistent breathing through your nostrils on a regular basis and during Power Programming.

1 Begin by pressing your finger against your right nostril and slowly inhaling through your left nostril for a count of 10 seconds.

2 Hold your breath for a moment and switch fingers so that you are now closing your left nostril.

3 Exhale through your right nostril for a count of 10 seconds.

4 Proceed by holding the left nostril and breathing in through the right. Exhale this time through the left.

5 Continue with this exercise alternating nostrils several more times.

Each of these breathing exercises will help you develop your relaxation response and prepare you to get maximum benefit from your Power Programming sessions.

THE RELAXATION RESPONSE IN ACTION

Now that you've mastered deep breathing, you're ready to take the next step to achieving total relaxation. I'm going to give you two of my favorite relaxation exercises. They will unlock the door to your subconscious mind and at the same time drain away stress and make you feel wonderfully peaceful.

The exercises I've selected are recorded on the Power Programming CD that comes with your book. You can listen to one or both of them. It really doesn't matter. The idea is for you to get a feel for this stuff. Practice either of these sessions every day for about a week. It will take you less than five minutes.

Now, it's time for you to open the CD sleeve bound into your book, keeping in mind that there are three things you need to have before you start listening to your CD:

1 An open mind
2 A quiet, comfortable place to sit or lie down
3 A comfortable position

First, let go of the buzz and clutter of your rational mind's thinking processes, and allow yourself to open up into a receptive frame of mind. Then, find a comfortable quiet place where there are no distractions. You can sit in a chair or recliner, lie on a couch, in your bed, or on a carpeted floor—whatever feels best. Once you are comfortably seated or lying down, place the CD in your player, press the start button, and close your eyes.

The first time you use your CD, listen to the introduction on Track 1 first. Then listen to either or both of the exercises: *Basic Relaxation* on Track 2, and *Floating Away Relaxation* on Track 3. For your reference, the CD script for each exercise is included below.

Basic Relaxation Exercise   CD TRACK 2

Begin by lying down in a comfortable position with one hand on your stomach. Close your eyes and take a deep belly-breath through your nostrils. Inhale ... and exhale ... very slowly. Take another deep breath ... inhale ... and exhale. Continue to breathe slowly and notice how relaxed you are beginning to feel already. Feel the relaxation each time you breathe. Imagine the oxygen spreading throughout your entire body, creating total relaxation.

Now imagine a single bright star up above in the sky of your mind ... far away in the distance in a beautiful black sky. Imagine slowly drifting toward the star like a slow-moving spacecraft. You feel calm and relaxed ... weightless as you move closer and closer to the star. Suddenly you reach the star and become engulfed by the healing, relaxing light ... a light that seems to consume your entire body and mind.... It makes you feel good.... It makes you feel relaxed.

Relax even more deeply now, enjoying that sense of timelessness ... that sense of tranquility ... Slowly you begin descending from the star ... bringing with you that warm, relaxed feeling ... and as you descend you drift deeper and deeper as you count down from 10 to 1:

10 ... deeper and deeper now ... 9 ... drifting deeper and deeper ... 8 ... 7 ... all the way down deep ... 6 ... 5 ... just letting go now ... 4 ... 3 ... deeper and deeper ... 2 ... and finally 1 ... deep, deep, deep into your relaxed subconscious.

Continue to enjoy this deep, subconscious experience for a moment and allow your mind to wander freely. [Pause for at least one minute.]

I am now going to count from 1 to 5, and when I reach the number 5 you will feel completely relaxed and in control. Each time you choose to do this kind of relaxation, you will be able to drift deeper:

1 ... coming out of that deep relaxed state ... 2 ... continuing to emerge now ... 3 starting to come back now ... 4 ... eyes are starting to open ... and 5 ... eyes are wide open, feeling refreshed and alert, and wonderful in every way.

Floating Away Relaxation Exercise   CD TRACK 3

Begin by taking a relaxing deep breath through your nostrils. Take another deep breath and feel the oxygen as it reaches the deepest recesses of your lungs.... Allow your breathing to return to normal now, and imagine that you are lying on a soft, comfortable raft floating on top of a calm, warm lagoon.... This is the most comfortable raft in the world.... Your feet and hands dangle, just barely touching the warm, blue water.... You can feel the sun beating down upon you as you enjoy drifting away on your comfortable raft. Take some time and soak in the pleasure and relaxation of this comfortable setting. [Pause for one minute.]

Imagine that this raft is magical.... It takes you to a place of total peace and tranquility without a care in the world.... Imagine it ... feel the relaxation.... Count down now from 5 to 1, and with each count, with each breath you take, imagine yourself becoming more and more relaxed: 5 ... more and more relaxed ... 4 ... 3 ... calm and relaxed ... 2 ... 1 ... very, very relaxed.

KEEP IN MIND...

Developing the relaxation response is the key to Power Programming. Only when your mind and body are truly relaxed can you enter your subconscious—your mental computer—and reprogram it for permanent weight loss. By practicing basic breathing and relaxation exercises, you condition yourself to be super-receptive to the Power Programming sessions you'll be introduced to in Chapter 8.

There are two additional and very important techniques used in Power Programming: *imagery* and *suggestion.* Read on to learn how the almost magical power of imagery and suggestion can help you to lose weight effortlessly—and to keep it off permanently!

CHAPTER 6

PROGRAMMING WITH IMAGERY AND SUGGESTION

Close your eyes. Imagine you're lying on a deserted white sand beach. Feel the sun shining down, warming your skin. Smell the salty tang in the air. Feel yourself sink into the sand as you feel totally at peace.

Now, imagine fishing on a golden lake, hearing nothing but the peaceful sounds of birds chirping as you enjoy the warm breeze caressing your skin.

As you read each of these descriptions, did you hear, smell, taste or feel the sensations I was describing? Your imagination is a powerful piece of mental software, and it's a key ingredient in effective Power Programming. In an instant, your imagination will let you close your eyes and go anywhere you want to go, experiencing all the feelings and sensations you choose. Imagery is the foundation of our thought processes, and fortunately it imposes no limitations. You can imagine yourself doing anything you want!

When you use imagery during your Power Programming sessions, you'll find that it will be critical in helping you change your eating and exercise habits. The better you can visualize or imagine something, the more effective your Power Programming sessions will be, so we'll spend some time in this chapter exploring the link between imagery and weight loss. Get ready for incredible, almost magical results!

IMAGES BECOME REALITY

Your subconscious mind can't tell the difference between the images you create when you close your eyes, and the images you actually experience as you go about your daily life. That's why world-class skiers spend so much time imagining the perfect ski run. In their minds, they practice over and over again the precise skiing movements they want to master. Studies have shown that that imagery can actually help their performance, because mental conditioning influences performance as much as physical conditioning. The better you can immerse yourself in an imagined situation, the better you'll be able to function in the same situation in real life.

Imagery and visualization elicit *real* feelings. That's why you feel such strong emotions when watching a movie or reading a book. And that's why a TV commercial showing a juicy flame-broiled burger and salty golden fries will cause you to crave fast food. It's also why you're going to use imagery to delete those junk food images and thoughts of junk food from your mental computer and replace them with healthier ones during your Power Programming sessions. These new images will help to put you in control of your eating habits and to slim down and stay that way forever. It's that simple!

As you use imagery during Power Programming, you'll be uploading self-control, motivation, and confidence to your mental computer. As a result you'll eat less, eat healthier foods, and exercise more, without even thinking about it. Using imagery is easy to do. It's built right into the Power Programming sessions on your CD.

Your subconscious mind responds to sensory stimulation. Here's an example of what I mean: The word "peach" creates an image in the mind. But in your subconscious mind it creates a much more vivid image if the peach is juicy, soft, and sweet, with a golden ripe color and a mouth-watering flavor. Vividly descriptive imagery that stimulates as many of your senses as possible has the greatest impact.

It's also true that different people respond differently to the various kinds of sensory stimulation. If you're not a visual person—meaning that you can't "see" an image when you close your eyes—you'll probably be more receptive to images related to smells or sounds. If you're a person who responds most strongly to feelings, you will probably be most receptive to images that focus on intense feelings or emotions. For example, if you are asked to imagine a soothing ball of light entering your body, you'll *feel* the light healing and relaxing all of the areas of your body. Or, if you're imagining an experience in the past when you felt really motivated or proud, you'll *feel* the experience vividly.

During Power Programming, you'll use imagery to picture yourself surrounded by all of the foods you normally crave, without a shred of desire or a yearning to eat any of them. To create the image in your mind, you might imagine sitting down for dinner perfectly content, with a sensible portion on your plate, and no inclination to go back for more.

Your Power Programming CD uses vivid sensory imagery to help you switch your cravings from junk foods to healthy ones and from huge portions to sensible servings. It will use imagery to stimulate your imagination. You'll see yourself sitting down for dinner and thoroughly enjoying a mouth-watering meal of wonderful healthy foods. You'll smell the aroma, see the tempting colors, and taste the delicious flavors of the nourishing food on your plate. That way you'll be programming your subconscious mind to desire these foods and seek them out. You'll imagine yourself eating slowly, becoming acutely aware of feeling full, and leaving food on your plate every time you have a meal. This will carry over to your everyday life where it will become automatic and easy for you to take control of your eating habits.

GETTING RID OF SPONTANEOUS IMAGES

There you are, lying in bed watching late-night TV and thinking about how much you need to get done at work the following day. Odds are you're going to start to feel stressed—and the image of a chocolate bar could easily pop into your head. You'll probably start to crave that chocolate bar. But once you begin using your Power Programming CD, your cravings will disappear, just as they did for my client Fran:

Fran thought she was going crazy because she couldn't stop thinking about food. She'd be going about her daily tasks when suddenly an image of a juicy hamburger or an ice cream cone would pop into her head. These nagging thoughts led to intense cravings and caused her to eat the wrong kinds of food all the time.

During her Power Programming sessions with me, Fran learned to gain control of the "food thoughts" that would pop into her mind as she went about her daily business. She did it by replacing old food thoughts with new ones which she programmed into her subconscious mind. They were filled with images of delicious, nutritious foods: a fresh crispy green salad or a huge, red, juicy tomato fresh from the garden. What's more, these healthy food thoughts occurred only when she was hungry. Fran imagined lunchtime approaching and envisioned herself eating vegetables and a few slices of juicy turkey breast or ripe fruits. And she saw herself with a smile on her face, feeling happy and satisfied. After just a few sessions, she had no problem avoiding junk food and she eventually lost 50 pounds. Not only was Fran at her thinnest, she was healthier overall and felt better and more energetic than ever before!

THINK YOURSELF THIN!

Remember, as I've said before, your mind can create virtually any image you want it to. If I asked you to close your eyes and imagine a green beach, you'd be able to do it, even though I don't think a green beach exists anywhere in the world. In much the same way, you can imagine how you'll look and feel as a thin person. With the Power Programming sessions on your CD, you'll be able to imagine yourself exercising every day with great eagerness, legs and feet moving gracefully, sweat beading down your forehead. You'll imagine yourself at a restaurant eating slowly, enjoying your food, and feeling 100 percent in control. You'll feel like a runaway train steaming straight through every obstacle, so that nothing can get in the way of your goals.

Positive affirmations are another extremely effective tool you can use to think yourself thin. They will help you reinforce the new images that you'll program into your mental computer as you use your Power Programming CD. Here are some examples; you can create more on your own:

The more I think thin, the more I am thin.

People are beginning to notice my slim, healthy body.

Nothing prevents me from being thin.

I am thin because I am always in control of my eating and exercise habits.

Use All Your Senses

The vividness of your images is critical to the success of Power Programming. That's why the Power Programming sessions on your CD are designed to utilize *all* of your senses. The more you involve senses in your imagery, the better your results. For example, if you imagine yourself at a wedding, you should hear the sounds of glasses clinking and people chattering. Smell the aroma of steamed vegetables and fresh fish or chicken and imagine being turned off by the sight and smell of high calorie, fatty foods. Taste and feel the texture of your favorite vegetables and healthy dishes. You'll be surprised at how much more receptive your subconscious will be when you involve sensory perceptions in your imagery.

If your goal is to start exercising, imagine hearing the sound of the morning alarm and awaking with a fury of motivation and dedication. See yourself with a smile on your face, running smoothly on your treadmill or jogging outdoors. Feel your feet as they land gently while you jog or walk. When you use all of your senses, your images become more realistic and your mind becomes more receptive to them. You'll find all of this and more on your CD.

Create End-State Imagery

On your Power Programming CD, I'll also ask you to create images in your mind of yourself looking and feeling as you will after you have achieved your weight loss goal. This is called *end-state imagery*. If your goal is to lose 25 pounds, for example, you'll imagine your pants falling loosely off your waistline. You'll imagine confidently looking into a mirror and seeing a slim, thin, strong and healthy image of yourself proudly grinning from ear to ear.

In one of the end-state imagery techniques you'll find on your CD, I'll ask you to look into a mirror and see a reflection of yourself six months from now, looking thin, muscular, and better than you've ever looked before. Then I'll help you reinforce this image in your subconscious by suggesting that from now on you are going to constantly see that reflection in your mind, and it is going to motivate you to stay on track until you achieve your goal.

Imagine Powerful Metaphors

Metaphors can be an extremely effective form of imagery. Here's one example of how you could use metaphors to create imagery: Imagine placing all of your cravings and bad eating habits in a cardboard box. Now, imagine dropping a wrecking ball on the box and seeing its contents turn to dust. Imagine breathing a deep sigh of relief. You feel free again; you feel ready to take charge. That's a metaphor! And it's worked with many of my clients.

Here's an example of an effective metaphor you can try if you tend to lie in bed at night worrying about daily hassles: As you lie in bed and the first troubling thought pops into your head (such as *I think I don't have enough money to pay the telephone bill this month*) imagine a large waste can beside your bed. Take that thought, and mentally drop the thought into the waste can. As each new worrying thought appears, mentally drop it into the can. Get rid of it.

Here's a third possibility: Imagine a beautiful garden surrounded by a white picket fence. By the gate, there is a large, sturdy oak tree.

As you approach the gate, take whatever worries you have and hang them on the tree. They'll be there waiting for you when you come back out of the garden. Just hang your worries, one by one, on the Worry Tree. Then open the gate and step into the beautiful, peaceful garden, and close the gate behind you.

You get the picture. Metaphors are extremely effective and that's why they are used frequently in all of the Power Programming sessions on your CD. But if you find yourself stressing about something, don't hesitate to try the simple metaphors I just mentioned, all on your own.

Change Your Feelings Using Imagery

On your Power Programming CD I'll also make use of imagery to help you change your mood or feelings. Not only will this help motivate you to lose weight, it will also make a big difference in your overall health and well-being. Here's how the technique works. I'll ask you to imagine yourself in your favorite place, either an actual place or an imaginary one. And I'll ask you to incorporate all of your senses into the scene to make it more powerful and effective.

If your favorite place is a forest, for example, you can imagine the ferns brushing against your legs, the sound of a stream gurgling in the distance, and the smell of the foliage all around. This type of imagery is very good at helping you transform tension and anxiety into feelings of peace and tranquility.

Once you've reached your peaceful state, it will be easy to access feelings like confidence, motivation, and discipline. You'll use these feelings during your Power Programming sessions to empower yourself to toss out the potato chips, eat smaller amounts, and feel ready to start exercising. That's what Andy did when he was trying to lose weight:

> Andy was 27 years old and knew it was time to get back in shape. He was a late-night snacker and, although he wanted to exercise, he could never motivate himself to get up

and go to the gym. Nor could he discipline himself to eat better. All that Andy needed was a mental tune-up to regain the motivation and discipline he lacked. During his Power Programming sessions, he imagined past events when he had demonstrated motivation and discipline. As he imagined these events, sure enough, the motivation and discipline re-emerged. Using Power Programming, he then linked these feelings with images of exercising and eating better.

Andy imagined himself waking up every morning feeling super-motivated and going to the gym. He imagined preparing healthy meals every day and having total control over snacking. His mind absorbed all of these images and he began to incorporate them into his daily life. After only six months, he shed all of the unnecessary fat on his body and replaced it with muscle. His motivation surged and he felt better than ever before.

POWER SUGGESTIONS

In addition to using imagery during your sessions, you'll also use what are known as power suggestions—the fuel that feeds Power Programming. Power suggestions are direct commands given to your subconscious mind during your sessions. They reinforce the imagery that you use to reprogram your subconscious. Remember, your subconscious listens and responds uncritically during Power Programming.

For example, *"I will wake up early every morning and exercise with great enthusiasm,"* is a power suggestion you'll find on your CD. Suggestions like this are very effective for reinforcing imagery. They will program your mind to start thinking this way all the time, without even realizing that you're doing it. They will influence everything you do.

In the same way that positive thoughts can empower you, negative thoughts can cripple you. The more you suggest to yourself, *"I don't have the time to exercise,"* or *"I just can't stay away from chocolate,"* the better the chances are that you'll continue with these behaviors. Every time you have a negative thought, you program your mind to think in a self-destructive way. But don't worry. Power Programming will have you switching from negative to positive very quickly. Here's how:

The Influence of Self-Talk

Most of the time you carry on a dialogue with yourself in your mind. You mentally talk to yourself almost non-stop—when you're in the car, in the office, doing laundry, putting the dishes away, or any of the many other things you do every day. I call this *self-talk* and it exerts an enormous influence on your behavior. If you've made plans to exercise, for example, your self-talk might convince you that you don't really need to exercise.

Just as negative self-talk works against you, positive self-talk exerts a powerful positive influence on your behavior. When Jennifer used Power Programming to make her self-talk positive, her weight gain problem vanished:

Jennifer had made a resolution to exercise regularly and to get up an hour earlier in the morning to do it. That commitment, coupled with the Power Programming strategies she had learned, transformed her self-talk from negative to positive, and that greatly influenced her ability to lose weight. Jennifer focused on how much she enjoyed exercising and how good it made her feel. She convinced herself that she would exercise with enthusiasm every day. She also visualized herself as thinner, healthier, and more confident.

On day one after Jennifer's first Power Programming session, her alarm went off in the morning and she immediately got out of bed without any urge to hit the snooze button—something she's never done before. She felt energetic and ready to go. Then, she concentrated on getting to the gym, burning calories, and losing 20 pounds. The following week, she felt even better, and she got up in the morning even more eagerly. What made her do it? Every day, throughout the day, she thought about how good she felt and she envisioned how she was going to look and feel as a much thinner woman six months down the road. Using Power Programming techniques she utilized these positive self-talk messages to reinforce her exercise commitment. Exercise is now a normal part of Jennifer's day. The positive thoughts, images, and rewards of exercise flood her mental computer every day, and she continues to watch the unwanted pounds melt away.

In Jennifer's case, positive self-talk reinforced her commitment to exercise and helped her overcome the nagging temptation to hit the snooze button and go back to sleep. And the more she held onto her vision of success, the stronger her positive self-talk became. Exercise and positive thinking became an automatic part of her daily routine, and she didn't even have to think about it.

If you embrace this kind of positive self-talk, you'll be on your way to the same results Jennifer achieved. Here's the kind of positive self-talk that will get results:

I am losing weight.

I have plenty of time to exercise.

I have control over everything I do.

I am excited about becoming slimmer and healthier.

Watch out for the kind of negative self-talk that will undo all your gains:

I wish I were more motivated.

I wish I could lose weight.

I'm just not an exerciser.

I just don't have the time.

Bob is a good example of someone who sabotaged himself with negative self-talk. If Bob had only known how, he could have stopped these problems right at the beginning by uploading positive self-talk messages to his subconscious. Here's what happened:

> Like Jennifer, Bob made a resolution to start exercising. He strenuously stuck with it for a couple of weeks, but sensed trouble because he knew he was going to be super-busy at work. He started telling himself that because he was busy, it would be okay to cut down on exercising.
>
> This was strike one for Bob. His negative self-talk was allowing viruses to invade his mental computer and disrupt his workout routine. One Sunday night, Bob decided that he would skip exercising the next Monday, but that he would definitely get back to it on Tuesday. However, he got home late Monday night and was worried that he'd be tired the next day. He said to himself, "If I skip exercising again on Tuesday, I'll get an extra 45 minutes of sleep."
>
> Strike two: Mental viruses started taking control of Bob's mental computer, as his negative self-talk weakened his motivation even more. In no time, the viruses were winning, as Bob's continuing excuses took him out of the exercise loop completely.
>
> Strike three: A full-blown mental computer crash. Bob fell back into his old routines and exercise became a distant thought in the back of his mind. Once again, regular exercise was far out of his reach.

Power suggestion and positive self-talk are about feeding your receptive mental computer with positive thoughts. When you use these techniques, you'll begin to go about your day believing in yourself and elevating your confidence.

Sending Only Positive Messages to Your Subconscious

Now that you understand how the subconscious accepts images and suggestions literally, it's important to know that it's not a good interpreter of the words *don't, won't,* and *not.* It's essential for you to avoid using negative words, as you'll notice I have done on your Power Programming CD. It's critical for you to identify the changes you *do* want, not the ones you *don't* want. For example, the suggestions you'll hear on your Power Programming CD will be something like this:

> I eat only when my body needs food and I'm comfortable eating small amounts.
>
> Not. . .
>
> I don't eat large portions.
>
> I don't eat when I'm not hungry.

Using negative words can confuse the subconscious. I'll give you an example of what I mean. If you play golf, you know that hitting the ball over a lake is nerve-wracking, because the last thing you want to do is take a penalty. Amateur golfers tend to do this often, largely because of their negative inner self-talk. Typically, what they say to themselves is: *I will NOT hit this shot into the lake.* Read that statement again and see what image comes to your mind. That's right, it creates a mental picture of the ball plunking into the lake!

Now say to yourself: *This shot is going to soar over the lake into the deep blue sky and land softly on the green.* Doesn't that create a much better image in your mind?

Here's another example. Right now, try as hard as you can to *not* think of the color of your eyes. The first thing you did was think about the color, wasn't it? Aren't you doing that right now, in fact, even though you're trying *not* to? Whenever you try not to do something, you must first think of the thing you don't want to happen. That's just the way your mind works.

If you want to change your eating habits, the same rules apply. A suggestion such as, *I eat slowly and am completely satisfied with smaller portions,* produces a mental image of self-control and eating less food. A suggestion such as *I don't eat large portions* or *I don't eat fatty foods,* produces a mental image of the offending foods. Stop reading for a moment and think about the difference between the two.

By sending only positive images and suggestions to your subconscious, you'll be able to take advantage of the remarkable power of this amazing tool for weight loss and any other goal you wish to achieve.

Post Power Suggestion

Another kind of power suggestion is known as a post power suggestion. A post power suggestion is a reminder or cue you program into your mind during your Power Programming sessions. It will kick in after the session is over, as you go about your day-to-day life. For example, during a session you might say, Every time I hear the sound of the refrigerator door open and close, I feel calm and in control. Thereafter, your subconscious will actually remind you of this and you will indeed feel calm and in control when the refrigerator door opens. Another easy post power suggestion is, Every time I feel a bit hungry, I will take a deep breath and feel calm and in control. Again, your subconscious will remind you to do this whenever you feel hungry. This is an extraordinary and very effective tool to use for weight loss. It works!

Using Power Affirmations

Power affirmations are the final building block in Power Programming. As stated earlier, an affirmation is a positive thought or statement that you repeat to yourself over and over again to reinforce a concept in your subconscious mind. Affirmations are similar to self-talk. The difference is in the repetition. It helps to program the affirmation into your subconscious where it will guide your desired thoughts and actions. Affirmations act to reinforce the imagery and power suggestions you'll use during Power Programming.

More often than not, you repeat negative statements to yourself on a daily basis, without even realizing it. You tell yourself that you can't do something, that you're too lazy, or that you're going to fail. The subconscious always accepts what you tell it. Once you start replacing negative self-talk with positive statements, and repeating them to yourself daily they become positive affirmations.

It is best to keep affirmations simple. A short sentence related to your Power Programming goals is enough. Something like, *"My eating habits are under my control at all times,"* is enough. It is the repetition, not the length, that is important. For the best results, do your power affirmations when you lie down to go to sleep at night. Close your eyes and say them to yourself 10 times. The more you concentrate, the more feeling you will put into your statement and the stronger and faster you'll see results. Here are some examples:

I am happy and strong.

I enjoy eating slowly and being in control.

Every day, in every way, I feel more and more
  motivated to succeed.

I am calm and cool in every situation.

I always feel alert and energetic.

I am successful in whatever I do.

KEEP IN MIND...

Your subconscious cannot tell the difference between the images and suggestions you create in your mind and the real ones you encounter in every day life. As a result, imagery and suggestion can be incredibly powerful tools for weight loss. When you power program your subconscious with the right images and suggestions, you'll find yourself automatically eating better and exercising more. Your excess weight will disappear without a struggle. Imagery and suggestion are most effective when you engage all of your senses.

Now that you understand how critically important imagery and suggestion are to Power Programming, you're ready to move on to Chapter 7 where you'll discover the secret to creating and sustaining another key to permanent weight loss—motivation.

But before you turn the page, try the brief imagery exercise that follows.

> ### *How to REACH Your Imagery Potential*
>
> You can summarize the most important aspects of imagery and suggestion with the acronym R-E-A-C-H.
>
> **R**elaxation   Having a relaxed mind and body enables you to use all of your senses during your imagery scenes. This will enhance the vividness of your images and increase their effectiveness.
>
> **E**xpediency   Be sure that the images you use are applicable to your needs and your goals. Be realistic about your goals so that you don't set yourself up for failure.
>
> **A**vailability   Be good to yourself by setting aside time to practice imagery and Power Programming. Keep your priorities focused and put your health and well-being at the top.
>
> **C**onsistency   Like any other skill, imagery takes practice. Be sure that you are consistent and that you practice regularly.
>
> **H**ighlight   Highlight imagery in your life and reinforce, reinforce, reinforce!
>
> Keep REACH in mind as you think about the incredible power of your subconscious to respond to images and suggestions.

IMAGERY IN ACTION

The best way for you to understand imagery is to actually experience it in action using your Power Programming CD, where you'll find a brief imagery exercise on Track 4. It's designed to help you use all of your senses to heighten the experience, and make it more powerful. Look at the exercise as a practice tool, a first step in training your mind for weight loss.

As soon as you have a little quiet time to yourself, slip the CD into your player, and find a comfortable place to sit or recline, just as you did when you practiced the relaxation exercises in Chapter 5. Lie back, breathe slowly and deeply, and then press the play button. That's all there is to it. For your reference, I'm including a script for the exercise below.

Brief Imagery Exercise   CD TRACK 4

Begin by slowly breathing in through your nostrils ... and exhaling through your mouth.... Take another deep breath and feel the air as it reaches the deepest part of your lungs.... Notice how quickly you are starting to relax already.

Now slowly count backwards from 10 to 1 and just let your mind drift and relax with each number:

10 ... slowly relaxing ... 9 ... more and more relaxed ... 8 ... feeling calm and relaxed ... 7 ... even deeper and more relaxed now ... 6 ... 5 ... deeper, relaxed ... 4 ... 3 ... just like that ... 2 ... and 1 ... completely relaxed....

Now, imagine that you are full of health and vitality.... Losing weight is the most important goal for you.... Imagine that you are always in control of your eating habits.... That's right, you are always in control of your eating habits....

Now imagine that it is Thanksgiving and you have just seated yourself to eat with family and friends.... Imagine a smile on your face.... You can hear the clinking of silverware and plates.... You can hear the sound of conversation circulating around the table.... You feel completely in control....

Now imagine your hunger feeling.... You feel slightly hungry, not starved ... and you realize exactly how much food your body needs.... You can smell the turkey and all the other food.... Imagine placing a reasonable amount of food on your plate.... Everyone else's plate is overflowing, but not yours ... not yours.... You are in control ... and that feels good ... that feels very good....

Now imagine sinking your teeth into a delicious piece of turkey and eating very slowly.... You always eat slowly ... and it makes you feel in control.... Imagine chewing your food slowly and thoroughly, enjoying it.... You notice that your hunger feeling has gone away and you stop eating ... you stop eating.... You stop long before you are full and that feels good.... You are always in control.

CHAPTER 7

UNLEASHING YOUR
MOTIVATION TO LOSE WEIGHT

Whatever your goal, the driving force that will ultimately bring you success is motivation. You probably think that people who are successful, wealthy, happy, or thin are lucky and fortunate. But the truth is, success has nothing to do with luck and good fortune. It's all about creating the motivation to achieve specific goals, and keeping that motivation alive.

A friend of mine is a world-class runner who competes in many races and marathons every year. He runs 60 miles a week to stay in shape, but when he's training for an upcoming event he pounds the pavement harder than usual, running 90 miles a week. How does he do it? By staying motivated. And he stays motivated by using Power Programming techniques to keep his mental software up to date and fully operational. If he didn't, he'd slip out of "the zone" and his motivation would eventually dwindle and disappear.

Motivation doesn't just materialize all by itself, out of thin air. You have to awaken it by programming your subconscious. And then you have to tightly hold onto it and reinforce it with your conscious mind, so it doesn't fade away. Just as with imagery and suggestion, you have to install new motivation software onto your computer—your subconscious mind—before you can get results.

Real, lasting motivation comes from your conscious and subconscious minds working together in a partnership to achieve the goal. Close your eyes and imagine yourself as vividly as possible achieving your goal—that's your conscious mind working. When you Power Program your mind for motivation, you reach your subconscious mind. Your subconscious mind will be ready for the programming, because your conscious mind has already been priming your subconscious for the Power Programming suggestions that are to come. The motivation created by this melding of your conscious and subconscious minds is permanent. It stays with you always.

Motivation creates a cycle of success. When you're on your way to reaching your goals, you feel much more powerful and purposeful, and that, in turn, strengthens your motivation. This is the first step in the cycle of success. If you're stuck in a sedentary lifestyle and you can't bring yourself to take the first big step, Power Programming will give you the thrust you need to begin.

Then, Power Programming will use imagery and suggestion to help you focus and maintain your motivation. Even if you manage to trigger just a flicker of motivation, it can be enough to start you off in the right direction. Once you've taken that first step, your motivation will increase naturally, and soon you'll be in cruise control, as your exercise and healthy eating become routine and you watch the pounds melt away!

In this chapter, you'll learn exactly how motivation works and how to apply it towards more healthy eating, exercise, and permanent, effortless weight loss.

Think Success

You've learned about the powerful tools of relaxation, imagery, and suggestion in previous chapters and you know how critically important they are to your success with weight loss. Through Power Programming, you'll use these tools to uncover the seeds of motivation lying dormant in your subconscious mind.

Maintaining motivation affects every goal you try to achieve. Let's take an example that's not related to weight loss. Let's say you have visions of becoming a financial planner. You'll have to hit the books and study long and hard for the demanding test. Just the thought of all the preparation and hard work, along with the insidious fear of failure, can prevent you from taking action because your conscious mind will put a damper on your efforts by analyzing everything and weighing the pros and cons. Soon, your conscious mind will be giving you reasons to procrastinate and then to put your financial planning goals on hold.

To awaken your motivation, you'll need to use your subconscious imagination to picture yourself several months from now with hoards of clients banging down your doors. These images will be very real to your subconscious and will help you achieve your goal of becoming a financial planner in exactly the same way that imagining yourself thin and healthy during your Power Programming sessions will help you lose weight.

You need to think very carefully about the statements you make to yourself—your self-talk—as you think about your goals. As you've already discovered, this self-talk will have a great influence on your ability to lose weight. For example, *"I'd like to lose weight"* is a much different statement from *"I'm going to lose weight."* The first example has no power. It briefly flickers through your mind and then burns out. The second example, however, is much stronger; it elicits conviction. The motivational force in your subconscious is hungry for these kinds of positive and powerful thoughts, and as you reinforce them with Power Programming, they will quickly take hold.

When you look into a mirror and say to yourself with conviction, *"It's time to lose weight,"* you will begin to envision yourself as slender, eating healthfully, and exercising. Your subconscious will be tapping you on your shoulder saying, *"Come on, let's go!"* But here's the problem: These visions are usually short lived. After they come, they lose their strength, and your motivation fades away. But once you begin using Power Programming, those fleeting thoughts and images will gain strength and fuel your motivation. Whether you want to lose weight or become a financial planner, the clearer and more powerful your thoughts and images are during Power Programming, the more realistic they become and the more you will build up the motivation you need to stick with your goals.

GET EXCITED!

The feeling of excitement is a driving force from your subconscious mind that gets you super-motivated, as my client Deborah discovered:

Deborah came for her first session, excited and hopeful about losing weight. She loved to eat fried chicken and potato chips, and she snacked late at night and never exercised. Deborah knew that if she was going to exercise, she had to do it before 7 A.M., her usual time for getting out of bed and getting ready for work. At one time in her life, she exercised regularly and enjoyed the way it made her feel and look, but now she was in a deep rut and couldn't get herself out. Each morning, she'd hit the snooze button instead of getting out of bed to exercise. Because Deborah was an intelligent, open-minded individual, she was an excellent candidate for Power Programming.

I guided her through a progressive relaxation exercise—just like the one in Chapter 5—and directed images and power suggestions to her subconscious mind. I asked her to imagine that she could break down her barriers and wake up feeling excited and ready to exercise. And I asked her to think back to past successful life experiences and re-experience all of the positive feelings associated with them. The wheels of her motivation began to turn. I suggested to her subconscious that the moment the alarm sounded, she would experience those positive and encouraging feelings.

Deborah silently repeated power affirmations (see Chapter 6) to herself every night to reinforce these feelings. Each morning she woke up and, without any resistance, she got on the treadmill. Later, she told me that every time she heard the alarm sound, she felt not only willing, but eager to exercise.

We also worked on improving Deborah's motivation to eat more healthfully. Again, she used imagery and suggestion to envision herself as in-control, slender, and in-shape. Some of the power suggestions I gave her were:

- You are always in control of what you eat.
- You are always in control of how you eat.
- Food is less and less important to you.
- Cravings for junk food and large portions are a thing of the past.

Deborah's subconscious grasped all of these images and suggestions, and within a few months she lost 45 pounds. Even though she was very open-minded and motivated, she was surprised at how quickly and easily she was able to lose so much weight.

Deborah learned to tap into her subconscious mind and use it to awaken her motivation and her excitement, and she refused to let anything break her motivation. She savored it and didn't allow it to fade.

Deborah knew consciously what she needed to do to lose weight. Everyone does. But she succeeded, where others fail, by Power Programming her subconscious mind to boost her excitement and keep her motivation alive. To keep the positive, motivating feelings fresh in her mind, she practiced 15 minutes of Power Programming just once or twice a week on a continuing basis. And she made sure to do her power affirmations every night before going to bed.

LISTEN TO YOUR SUBCONSCIOUS

If you suddenly feel a tweak of motivation to lose weight, don't just take it for granted. Savor it! Grab hold of it tightly before it fades away. Your subconscious is trying to reach out to you, and you need to grasp the opportunity. Look at it like this: I'm sure you've had vivid dreams that seemed very real. You wake up and remember every detail, and then you fall back asleep and forget the dream ever happened. Now, if you had used Power Programming and asked your subconscious to remind you to write down the details of your dreams, you wouldn't forget them; you'd remember them before they slipped away. It's the same with motivation. If you ask your subconscious to bring your motivation to the forefront so that you always have access to it, it will always be there, ready to support you.

As an avid runner, I'm constantly aware of my motivational levels. Many nights in the past, I'd be driving home from work and feel tempted to skip my exercise routine even though I had made a commitment to myself earlier that day. Most of the time, my conscious mind would end up convincing me to skip my exercising. In other words, my conscious and subconscious minds were on two different pages. But when I began to practice Power Programming, I was able to overcome and eliminate conscious temptations and excuses—viruses that attempted to invade my mental computer. I trained my subconscious to instantly become aware of these sabotaging, conscious thoughts and to redirect them to the feelings I experience when I'm motivated—feelings like confidence and self-control.

MAKING MOTIVATION AUTOMATIC

Have you ever been hit with a blast of motivation when you didn't expect it? Maybe you weren't eating such healthy meals, and you suddenly felt determined to change. This new-found motivation didn't just happen. Somewhere along the line you tweaked your subconscious mind a little bit, without realizing it, and made it understand that you were fed up with being fat. Now all you need to do is feed the motivation and reinforce it with Power Programming techniques.

When you generate thoughts of eating healthfully and exercising regularly, if you burden them with excuses, temptations, and other viruses, you're not going to feel very motivated. Let's say you've made a commitment to avoid late night cookies and milk. After a long day, you cook dinner, get the kids ready for bed, prepare their lunches for the next day and after they are in bed, you finally sit down and relax. You surf through the channels for something to watch on TV. The chocolate chip cookies in the cabinet and the creamy milk in the refrigerator start to creep into your mind. Your conscious mind starts to weigh the pros and cons. The temptations increase and before you know it you're saying to yourself, "Just one more night of milk and cookies won't make a difference." Before long, you're gobbling down high-calorie cookies and guzzling milk, and once again your commitment is in tatters. What you need to do is train your subconscious to catch those thoughts and redirect them to stop the cravings and build motivation to stick to your commitment.

Now, imagine taking all of the benefits of motivation and self-control, supercharging them, and plugging them into your mental hard drive. This is exactly what Power Programming will do for you. Your subconscious will take this arsenal of positive thinking and use it to wipe out the conscious impulses that lead you to failure. Remember, you respond to your thoughts, and when your thoughts are full of passion, power, and belief, you can bring yourself to do just about anything. That's exactly what happened with Jane:

Jane was 200 pounds overweight and had never exercised a day in her life. She was critical of herself and had a rather cynical personality. We agreed that exercising had to be her priority. She and her husband had purchased a treadmill that they never used, but Jane claimed that she couldn't bring herself to exercise in the cold, dark basement where the treadmill was located. She also convinced herself that because she was so heavy, she would only be able to walk slowly and it wouldn't accomplish anything. Her negative self-talk was convincing her to avoid the very thing that would help her solve her weight problem.

During our first Power Programming session, Jane imagined herself going to the basement, feeling disciplined and motivated. She then linked these qualities to a scene six months later, where she looked thinner and felt great. Then at our next session, Jane told me things hadn't gone well. She had only exercised six days that week and was very disappointed for missing a day! Remember now, this is someone who never exercised before. Her mind accepted everything we did in the first session so literally that exercising became a normal and expected thing for her. Missing one day seemed like a lot.

Jane completely changed her eating habits, too. She used to eat a lot of snack foods and she overate during meals. Using Power Programming, she deleted the impulse to snack from her mental computer. Without any effort, she stopped snacking and began eating sensible portions. After re-programming her subconscious mind, her new weight loss plan felt normal and effortless, and her thoughts quickly shifted in a positive direction.

Three months after our final session, Jane was still exercising six times a week and eating healthfully, and her weight continued to come off. Jane lost 35 pounds those first couple of months and was down 120 pounds the last time I spoke with her.

Motivation is the catalyst to change. You don't need to have the motivation of a marathon runner to be successful. All that's required is to spark some of the motivation in your mental computer, and then use Power Programming as your ticket to success.

KEEP IN MIND...

You already have motivation within yourself, and by accessing your subconscious you can unveil it. When you use Power Programming to visualize yourself achieving your goal, you will start to notice your motivation increasing. When you fortify that positive image with passion and success, your motivation will grow and flourish. The weight will start coming off, and you will become healthier day-by-day.

Now that you understand all about Power Programming and how you can use it to fat-proof yourself permanently, it's time to move on to Part Three, which will prepare you for listening to your CD and beginning your first Power Programming session! Before you move on, though, try out the following motivation exercise for priming your mental computer to achieving your weight loss goals! It's included on your Power Programming CD.

JUMPSTARTING YOUR MOTIVATION

Find a quiet place where you can lie back, relax, and listen to this exercise on your CD player. It will start your motivational juices flowing and demonstrate what a powerful difference that can make. The exercise combines deep breathing, imagery, and suggestions, and is similar to the imagery exercise in Chapter 6, but this time it focuses specifically on motivation.

Once you're comfortable, begin breathing slowly and deeply and then press the play button on your CD player, lie back, and close your eyes. For your reference, a script of the exercise follows.

Brief Motivation Exercise   CD TRACK 5

Begin by taking a deep, slow breath.... Count slowly backwards from 5 to 1: ... 5 ... 4 ... feeling very comfortable and relaxed ... 3 ... drifting and dreaming ... 2 ... more and more relaxed now ... 1 ... feeling peaceful and relaxed....

Imagine now that you have lost the amount of weight you no longer want or need.... You see a thin and slim image of yourself and you feel so happy and so secure ... feeling great and looking good.... Your family and friends all praise and admire you.... You feel driven.... You feel unstoppable....

Feel that motivation now ... feel it.... See that thin you.... You are more motivated and in control than you've ever been.... ... ... Nothing gets in your way.... ... ... Feel that motivation.... ... ... See that thin you.... See the clothes hanging loosely from your body.... Enjoy the admiration and comments you get from everyone you know.... Really feel those good, powerful feelings....

You are in control....

Imagine now that you have made a resolution to begin exercising ... and you have those powerful, motivating feelings within you right now.... Just imagine waking up to the sound of your alarm.... You can hear the sound of it right now.... The first thing you think of is that image of the thin you ... that vivid image ... ... the true you. Any time you hear that alarm from this point on you will see that vivid image of the thin you in your mind ... and you will bounce right out of bed.... ... ... That's right ... you'll bounce out of bed....

PART THREE

Your 3-Week
Power Programming
Weight Loss Program

CHAPTER 8

USING YOUR POWER
PROGRAMMING WEIGHT LOSS CD

Now you're ready to begin losing weight using my simple Power Programming techniques. On your CD, you'll find three complete Power Programming sessions. You should devote one week to each session, for a total of three weeks.

For the first week, you'll focus on Track 6, *Cracking The Code To Your Eating Habits*. Listen to just this session, once a day for an entire week.

For week two, you'll move on to Track 7, *Unlocking Your Motivation and Self-Control*. Again, you'll repeat this session every day for the full week.

For week three, you'll finish with Track 8, *Strengthening Your New Skills*. Listen to this session daily for the final seven-day period.

That's all there is to it. In less than 20 minutes a day, the complete three-week program will bring amazing results. But before you begin listening to the CD, take a look at the steps involved in Power Programming so you'll be able to get the most out of each session. Each Power Programming session progresses through 5 steps, but you won't notice these steps while you're listening, because they will flow naturally for you:

Step 1: Log on to your mental computer using your relaxation
        password
Step 2: Go deeper to access your computer's command center
        (your subconscious)
Step 3: Download weight loss imagery software

Step 4: Turbocharge your computer with forceful commands

Step 5: Log off and exit to your conscious state

STEP 1: LOG ON TO YOUR MENTAL COMPUTER USING YOUR RELAXATION PASSWORD

Relaxation is the password that allows you to log on to your mental computer. In this first stage of Power Programming, your mind and body will become profoundly relaxed, giving you access to your computer's command center—your subconscious mind—and making it receptive to reprogramming. In this step, Power Programming will lead you into a very deep state of relaxation and create the *relaxation response* described in Chapter 5. You're likely to experience some of the physical signs of deep relaxation. These include tingling in the hands or feet, flickering and fluttering of the eyelids, a sensation of heaviness or lightness, a need to swallow, and time distortion. These are normal and are good indicators that your mind and body are relaxed and that you are tapping into your subconscious.

When your mind and body are relaxed, the conscious part of your mind, the part that critiques and analyzes all of your actions and decisions, will become far less intrusive, and your subconscious will take over as the dominant state of mind. In this state of mind you'll become super-receptive to all of the weight loss images and commands that you want to program into your subconscious mind. Just like any other computer, your subconscious mind will accept the programming unconditionally.

Another important part of this first stage of Power Programming is stress reduction. Don't forget, whenever you are deeply relaxed, it is impossible to be stressed. As you continue to practice Power Programming relaxation techniques, you'll find that your body achieves a natural relaxation response that carries over from your Power Programming sessions into the stressful situations in everyday life. When you're feeling stressed, rather than reaching for a bowl of super-high-calorie ice cream, you'll automatically slow down, relax, breathe deeply, and calm yourself instead. All of this will happen naturally as a result of Power Programming.

STEP 2: GO DEEPER TO ACCESS
YOUR COMPUTER'S COMMAND CENTER

In Step 2, you'll deepen your relaxation in order to connect directly with the command center of your mental computer. With a direct line of communication, your subconscious will become ultra-receptive to Power Programming. As you become more experienced, your mind will become so accustomed to this deep state of relaxation, it will be all you need to tap into your mental command center. The easiest method for deepening your level of relaxation is to simply count from 10 to 1. With each number you count, you'll feel yourself going more and more deeply into a state of complete relaxation.

STEP 3: DOWNLOAD WEIGHT LOSS
IMAGERY SOFTWARE

Now you're at a point where you can actually reprogram your computer's command center. You'll be able to uninstall old software you no longer need and replace it with brand new imagery software. Think of your Power Programming CD as a software CD-ROM packed with the latest, state-of-the-art software updates. With it you can create vivid scenes that will help you avoid high-calorie, high-fat foods, control your eating habits, and exercise with passion and fury. Best of all, these changes in your everyday habits and choices will happen automatically. You won't even need to think about it.

As you read in Chapter 6, these powerful images will help your mind paint pictures of the sights, sounds, smells, and tastes that will help you achieve your weight loss goals. You'll also discover hidden emotional treasures, like self-control, confidence, and motivation. While you're listening to your CD, these images will feel very realistic. You'll feel as if the scenes you are imagining are actually happening and you'll enjoy how it feels to be completely in control.

You'll be amazed that your creative subconscious is so strong and active. Many people experience imagery scenes so realistic, they act as if the scenes are actually happening. For example, someone who imagines eating a delicious, juicy piece of fruit will frequently salivate and swallow. This type of reaction demonstrates the power of the mind and the imagination, and it's very likely to occur during your session.

STEP 4: TURBOCHARGE YOUR COMPUTER WITH FORCEFUL COMMANDS

Now you're ready to turbocharge the imagery software you've just installed in your computer. In Step 4 you'll give your subconscious direct commands for losing weight. These commands can be compared to configuring your software and telling it what to do. At this stage your subconscious is super receptive. It will accept these commands without question, and you will find yourself acting upon the commands without even thinking.

By the time you get to this step, your subconscious mind will be ready for suggestions that are forceful and direct. As your control becomes firmer, you'll begin to notice a newfound sense of power over feelings of hunger, exercise, and thoughts about food and situations in which food is present. For some people, the feelings of control and discipline have been buried for so long, it feels magical and incredibly empowering to bring them to the surface again.

STEP 5: LOG OFF AND EXIT TO YOUR CONSCIOUS STATE

Returning to your conscious state of mind is very simple. The standard technique is counting from 1 to 5. I've had many clients struggle to open their eyes fully at this point because they were enjoying the experience so much! The moment you "come back," you're going to feel refreshed and alert. You'll feel as if every ounce of stress has drained away, renewing your outlook on life!

LISTENING TO YOUR POWER PROGRAMMING SESSIONS

Now that you know what to expect, you're ready to start the three-week Power Programming weight loss program. As I stated earlier, the CD that comes with this book contains three Power Programming sessions, one for each week of the program. Each session lasts less than 20 minutes. Written reference copies of the scripts for all three sessions are included at the end of this chapter.

Now, to help you get started, here are step-by-step guidelines for each of the three weeks:

Week 1: Cracking The Code to Your Eating Habits

Find a comfortable place where you can relax without being interrupted. Perhaps you have a private sanctuary downstairs in the basement or maybe in an upstairs bedroom. I like to listen to my Power Programming sessions during my lunch break at work. I usually take a ride in my car, park in a peaceful spot, recline the seat, and pop in my CD. If you decide to do this, you'll not only find that it helps you lose weight, you'll also be invigorated when you head back to work.

Once you have found your little hideaway, all you have to do is make yourself comfortable, pop in the CD, select Track 6, press the play button, lie back, and close your eyes. Listen to Track 6 every day for 7 days. You'll move on to Track 7 the following week.

Week 2: Unlocking Your Motivation and Self-Control

By this time, you've listened to the first Power Programming session for one full week. Your eating habits are improving, and your confidence is building. Now it's already time to begin your second week of Power Programming.

Once again, go to your comfortable hideaway, put your CD into the player, select Track 7, lie back, close your eyes, and get ready to take your confidence to another level, a level that will have you feeling super-motivated and in control in no time.

Week 3: Strengthening Your New Skills

Two weeks of power programming have already flown by, and now you're ready to graduate to Week 3 and the third and final Power Programming session on your CD. So, return to your hideaway, select Track 8, press play, lie back, and enjoy. Track 8 will reinforce all of the Power Programming that has taken place in the previous two weeks. As before, you'll listen to this track every day for seven days.

When Week 3 is over, you're finished! During this time, you've connected with your subconscious—your mental computer. You've uninstalled the virus-infected software that caused you to gain weight and thwarted your weight loss efforts. And you've installed brand new self-empowerment software that redefines who you are and what you are able to do.

After Week 3—Then What?

After you complete the three-week program it's important for you continue listening to Power Programming sessions, but you don't have to listen to the CD every day, and you don't have to listen to the Power Programming sessions in any particular order. You can now listen to any session you want, whenever you choose.

You may find that you enjoy Power Programming so much that you'll want to create your own personalized Power Programming sessions and record them on a cassette player or a portable media player. By recording personalized sessions, you can target your own individual goals or focus extra effort to overcome a specific hurdle. Or you may want to do it just for the sake of variety. You are the pro now, and the choice is yours. The Special Section at the end of this book gives you advice for recording your own Power Programming sessions, and it even includes two scripts that I created with personalization in mind.

Whether you stick with the Power Programming sessions on the CD, or record your own, here's a *very important* word to the wise: Don't stop completely! I recommend listening to at least one Power Programming session weekly—mine or your own—after you have completed the 3-week program. That way, you won't lose sight of your weight loss focus, you'll keep the momentum going, and you'll guarantee that each and every pound you lose will never come back. Ever!

THE POWER PROGRAMMING SCRIPTS

For reference purposes, here are written scripts for each of the three Power Programming sessions recorded on your CD:

Session 1: Cracking the Code to Your Eating Habits   CD TRACK 6

You are about to tap into the amazing power of your subconscious mind to help yourself achieve the results that you desire. Close your eyes and begin by taking a deep, relaxing breath of air, inhaling through your nostrils and exhaling through your mouth.... Take another relaxing deep breath of air and feel the air as it flows through your entire body and relaxes it....

Focus your attention on your forehead now.... Tighten your forehead area for several seconds.... Now relax your forehead.... Feel the relaxation as it fills your forehead area.... ... ... Now tighten your cheek muscles and hold for several seconds.... ... Let go and relax your cheeks now ... feel the relaxation as it fills both cheeks.... ... Direct your attention around your mouth area now.... Tighten your lips and your mouth and hold for several seconds.... ... ... Let go and feel the relaxation as your entire mouth area relaxes completely. Make sure that your teeth are parted slightly.... That's right.

Now, focus your attention on the area around your shoulders and neck.... Tighten this area and hold it for several seconds.... ... ... Now release the hold and feel the relaxation as it flows through your entire neck and shoulder area, getting rid of any tension there....

As your neck, shoulders, and facial area continue to relax, I would like you to bring your attention to your arms.... Tighten your biceps and hold for several seconds.... ... ... Let go now, and allow your biceps to relax completely.... ... ... Tighten your triceps now, those muscles in the back of your arms, and hold.... ... Release your hold and feel your triceps relax ... nothing to do but relax.... Just allow the tension to melt away completely....

Bring your attention to your forearms now and hold those muscles tight for a few seconds.... Let go and allow your forearms to relax.... Clench your fists very tightly for several seconds.... Feel the discomfort ... and allow your hands to relax now.

Now, bring your attention to your back muscles for a moment.... Squeeze together your shoulder blades and hold for several seconds.... ... ... Let go and feel the relaxation as it spreads throughout your entire back region.... Feeling so good and so relaxed....

Focus now on your stomach muscles.... Take a deep breath and hold it. Now tighten your stomach muscles for five seconds. [Pause five seconds.] Release your hold as you exhale and feel the stress and tension in your stomach fade away.... Feel the relaxation in the stomach area.... ... ... Feel it.

Bring your attention to your legs now.... Tighten your upper leg muscles (quadriceps and hamstrings) and hold for several seconds ... that's right.... Let go and allow relaxation to fill your entire upper leg area.... Tighten your calf muscles now and hold for several seconds.... ... ... Let go and allow the relaxation to fill this area as well.... ... Now clench your toes lightly and hold for several seconds.... ... ... Release the hold and allow relaxation to take over your feet.... Allow your entire body to continue to relax, feeling so comfortable and so completely relaxed.... That's right.

Many people experience certain feelings as they drift into that relaxed trance-like state.... ... Some people experience a numb feeling or a tingling feeling, usually in the hands or feet and sometimes in the arms and legs ... and other people experience both a numbness and a tingling sensation.

Some people experience a feeling of lightness, while others may experience a feeling of heaviness.... If you were to have that light feeling, you would feel as if you were just floating above your couch or chair, barely touching it.... And if you were to have that heavy feeling, you would feel as if you were just sinking into your seat, deeply, with your shoulders sagging.

Another interesting thing that some people experience while in this relaxed state is a need to swallow because when you are relaxed like this, your salivary glands become dry ... and if you have that need to swallow right now, it is perfectly OK to do so.... ... ...

Some people notice that while in this relaxed state, their eyelids seem to relax in their sockets causing the eyelids to flicker and flutter very lightly ... ... that's right.... ... ...

If you have experienced any of these sensation then it indicates your willingness and your readiness to allow yourself to go into this deep, trance state ... ... and going into this state is very gradual, and in a few moments, you're going to go even deeper.... ... ... But before you go deeper, I would like for you to use that powerful imagination of yours again.... ... ... I want you to imagine a soft, cuddly cloud that you seem to melt into.... ... ... This cloud can be any color you choose.... ... ... This is the most comfortable cloud in the whole world.... This cloud is going to take you to a very special place in your life.... It can be a real place or an imagined place ... a place where you're happy, confident, motivated, safe, and secure.... Just allow this soft relaxing cloud to take you to that very special place, and as I'm counting you'll drift deeper and deeper.... ... ...

10 ... going deeper and deeper now ... 9 ... just drifting and relaxing ... 8 ... 7 ... deeper and deeper ... 6 ... just ... letting go ... now ... 5 ... 4 ... all the way down deep ... 3 ... 2 ... and finally ... 1 ... deep, deep, and deeper....

The next time you want to reach a deeply relaxed state like this, all you need to do is take a deep breathe, tighten your stomach muscles for 5 seconds and exhale slowly, allowing all stress and tension to drift away.

Your mind is now relaxed and completely open and receptive to all of the beneficial suggestions and images that I am about to give to you.

Now that you have reached a very deep and relaxed state, your subconscious mind is ready to help you achieve any goal ... ... including your goal to lose weight.... ... ... The following images and suggestions are going to seal themselves in the deepest part of your subconscious, making weight loss easy and effortless.... ... ...

The first thing that I would like for you to do now is to imagine that you have already lost the amount of weight you no longer want, need, or desire.... ... ... You see an image of yourself that looks exactly how you want to look and feels slim and trim ... ... and you are imagining that you have maintained this weight loss without any struggle.... ... ... Because your subconscious is open and receptive, you can begin to see and feel what it is like to be slimmer, thinner, and in shape.... ... ... Your subconscious mind will now act on this slim healthy image and it now becomes your reality. From now on this image will always be present in your mind and you will easily and effortlessly allow yourself to lose the amount of weight you no longer want or need.

Imagine waking up to a perfect day now ... ... perfect because today you have turned the page.... ... ... Today is the first day of the rest of your life ... ... the first day of health and total self-control.... ... ... From this moment on, you change negative eating habits into good ones ... ... and you do this easily and effortlessly.... ... ... Your subconscious now rejects the foods that are harmful to your body and soul.... ... ... That's right, your mind now rejects all of those foods that you know are bad for you.... ... ...

I'd like for you to imagine being in a situation where, in the past, you would have felt vulnerable to poor eating.... ... ... Maybe you're at a restaurant, or a party, or a work function.... ... ... Whatever the situation is, you see all of those unhealthy foods and large portion sizes right in front of you.... ... ... You see the sweets.... ... ... You see the foods that are loaded with carbohydrates. You see the snack foods and junk foods.... ... ...

Now, something interesting is happening to you.... ... ... You look at these foods in complete disgust, and as you are imagining doing this ... ... all of these foods that you know are harmful violate your new health ... ... your new self-control.... ... Because of this, you take your arm and sweep it across the table, removing all of those harmful foods ... ... and as they crash on the floor, they are removed from your thought altogether.... ... ... From this point on, your subconscious mind rejects and detests these foods.... ... ... You find it absolutely effortless to avoid these foods, and that makes you feel good ... ... that makes you feel good.... ... ...

Now, you look at that empty table ... ... and you place all of the healthy, colorful foods that you like on it.... ... ... You see your favorite vegetables and fruits spread across the table.... ... ... You see all of the healthy, fresh foods on that table and you desire these foods ... ... you salivate looking at them.... ... ... Just the thought of fattening, large portions and junk foods makes your stomach turn.... ... ... You never want those foods again.... ... ... You are happy knowing that you can easily reach for all of the healthy foods that you know are good for you.... ... ... You are happy filling your body and mind with this kind of health and nurturing.

You feel proud that you have the control and power within you to relax and make healthy choices ... ... and you do it effortlessly ... ... as effortless as it is to feel as relaxed as you feel right now. You are a new, self-controlled person and you know that you can apply this same mental strength to anything, including exercising ... ... making exercise a part of your regular routine the same way you make healthy eating a part of your regular routine.

You now have new ways to deal with your old habits. You eat the foods you like, the foods that are healthy for you.... ... ... You are always in control of what you eat and how much you eat no matter where you are.... ... ... You apply this same level of self-nurturing and self-control to exercise, making exercise an easy part of your regular routine.... ... ... You desire these changes and you achieve them easily and effortlessly. Your subconscious absorbs all these suggestions. You feel wonderful and you can begin to feel that new, healthy power and energy that flows through you. You feel confident and powerful, and these confident, powerful feelings grow stronger and stronger every day. And you continue to relax now.

I am now going to count from 1 to 5, and when I reach the number five, you will open your eyes fully, feeling completely refreshed and alert: ... 1 ... coming out of the that deep trance state feeling wonderful in every way, feeling completely confident and in control in every way ... 2 ... continuing to emerge now, feeling wonderful in every way ... 3 ... starting to come back now ... 4 ... eyes are starting to open ... and 5 ... eyes are now wide open, and you are feeling refreshed and alert and wonderful in every way.

Session 2: Unlocking Your Motivation and Self-Control   **CD TRACK 7**

As you sit or lie down comfortably, find a spot or an object that is just above eye level and focus on it. Make sure to move only your eyes and not your entire head as you focus on the spot or object.... ... ... Allow your eyes to just rest there, focusing on that spot, and continue to relax.... ... ...

And as you continue to relax, you may begin to notice some slight changes occurring.... ... Perhaps your eyes are getting blurry and it is difficult to focus.... That's fine.... Maybe your eyes are getting very tired and it is becoming increasingly difficult to keep them open as you focus on that one spot.... Perhaps a part of you tries not to pay attention to those changes as you use all of your effort to hold your eyes there on that one spot, as you use all of your effort to hold your eyes there.... ... ...

And after a while, you might begin to notice the effort it takes to try not to pay attention to those sensations ... the blurriness ... the heaviness of the eyes ... or the way the spot seems to dance around and expand in shape, size, and color.... ... ...

And your eyes now become more and more tired ... more and more heavy.... ... ... There is more and more of a burning sensation than just a little while ago when you first started ... and perhaps your eyes begin to tear a little and want to close ... or blink ... or want to remain closed.... That's right.... Because we all know what it feels like when the eyes get tired ... as the mind and body relax.... We've all fallen asleep in front of the television ... that drifting barely awake feeling. We all know that it would be so much more comfortable to just allow the eyes to close, if they haven't already ... because after some time they are very tired and very heavy ... very tired and very heavy.... They seem to close automatically ... all by themselves ... your eyes can close.... And as they close—or if they are already closed—you can now begin to feel that tired, heavy, relaxed feeling.... That feeling spreads throughout the entire body ... the face ... the neck and shoulders ... the back ... and right into the legs and feet....

And because your entire body can be so very relaxed, the mind becomes relaxed as well ... and your inner, subconscious mind can begin to pay more attention as your conscious mind just drifts off somewhere else.... And as your mind and body continue to relax and as you continue to drift deeper and deeper, your subconscious can hear everything I say to you.

I'd like for you to imagine now that you are standing at the top of a beautiful old Victorian staircase. You can smell the newly refinished wood.... This staircase is very safe and has a beautiful banister running down it.... In a moment I am going to ask you to move slowly down this wonderful staircase as I count from ten to one, and as I count, you will move slowly down the staircase and go deeper and deeper into that trance state. Imagine taking your first step down ... 10 ... going deeper and deeper, safe and secure ... 9 ... feeling the smooth banister as you slowly drift down deeper ... 8 ... more and more relaxed, deeper and deeper ... 7 ... 6 ... just gliding and floating ... 5 ... 4 ... just letting go now ... 3 ... that's right ... 2 ... and finally ... 1.... You are now at the bottom of the staircase and your mind is completely relaxed and open to receiving all the helpful and beneficial suggestions that I am about to give to you.

Because you are now completely in control of your eating habits, I'm going to give you some more images and suggestions that are going to reinforce everything you've experienced so far ... multiplying your motivation and self control like never before....

Everything you are about to hear is going to allow you to take complete control over your eating and exercise habits.... ... ... These suggestions are going to seal themselves into the deepest part of your subconscious, giving you more motivation and self-control than you've ever had, making eating normal portions of food second nature to you.

Imagine that you have just arrived at your favorite restaurant with friends. It is a Saturday evening and the restaurant is packed.... ... ... The hostess seats your party and you are enjoying the company of your friends.... ... ... A basket of bread is placed on the table as you converse and laugh with your friends.... ... ... It is very enjoyable to be with the people you are with.... ... ... You are hungry ... ... but you are also very relaxed, almost as relaxed as you feel right now.... ... ... You take a piece of the bread and you tear it in half, and this is perfectly fine.... ... ... Perhaps you place a touch of butter or olive oil on the bread ... ... and you eat that half piece of bread very, very slowly.... ... ... You chew and swallow extremely slowly and that feels good.... ... ... From now on, every time you sit down to eat, you automatically remember to eat ... very ... ... slowly.... ... That's right, you eat very ... ... slowly ... ... and your mind accepts this suggestion.... ... ... You finish your small piece of bread and it feels as if it took an eternity to finish it ... ... and you continue to converse, and you become very aware of how everyone else is eating.... ... ... Some of the people you're with have already had two or three pieces of bread ... ... and knowing that further enhances your feeling of self-control.... ... ... That further empowers you.... ... ...

A feeling of peace and calmness sweeps over you ... a feeling of excitement.... ... ... It feels good being so in control.... ... ... You are always in control of how you eat and you enjoy eating slowly.... ... ... In the past, you probably would have been on your third piece of bread by now, but not anymore, not you.... ... ... It just feels right to eat less ... ... it feels very normal for you. Your subconscious mind accepts this completely.... ... ...

Your friends have decided to order several appetizers for everyone to share at the table.... ... ... Imagine these appetizers. They can be any appetizers that come to your mind first.... ... You are very aware of your hunger feeling, and you take a small piece of an appetizer ... ... and you eat very slowly, almost in slow motion.... ... ... You savor every bite.

Several minutes have gone by and all of the appetizers are gone, and that makes you feel good.... ... ... You've eaten a minute amount and you feel even more in control ... ... effortlessly.... ... ... You notice how some of your friends have shoveled the appetizers into their mouths and you enjoy knowing that you no longer eat that way.... ... ... It feels wonderful to be in such control of your behavior.... ... ... You feel good ... ... you feel confident ... ... you feel empowered.... ... ...

One of your friends turns to you and says, "Are you alright, you're barely eating." And you say to him, "I'm just fine. I'm completely satisfied. Things couldn't be any better.".... ... Your friends look bewildered ... ... and this further fuels your self-discipline and self-control.... ... ...You know the secrets that they don't know.... ... ... You feel the power of your mind ... ... the power of self-control.... ... ... You know how to eat normally now, to eat less and to stop long before you're full.... ... ... You never want to feel full again, because when you're full it means that you have eaten entirely too much.... ... ... You love your newfound self-control. Your subconscious accepts all of this and it is your new reality.

The server now brings out the entrées.... ... ... Again, you pay close attention to your hunger and you realize that your hunger feeling is almost gone completely.... ... ... Once again you take slow, deliberate bites and you do so easily and automatically.... ... ... You look around and notice that everyone has finished eating including you. But for you there is something different.... ... ... You are the only one who still has food on the plate.... ... ... You leave half or more of your entrée on the plate and you ask for it to be wrapped so you can take it home with you ... and that feels good. That feels normal to you.... ... ... Your friends look at you again with that bewildered expression ... ... and there is a smile on your face.... ... ...

The server arrives some time later and takes the dessert order.... ... ... You order no dessert because you are not hungry ... ... and that feels fine ... ... that feels normal.... ... ... The rest of the table looks at you in amazement. They have all ordered dessert ... ... but not you ... ... not you.... ... You enjoy their admiration.... ... ... Another friend turns to you and asks, "Can you tell me how you did this tonight?" You smile and chuckle and say, "I have learned how to Power Program my mind."

Your subconscious mind accepts all of these images and suggestions.... ... ... You leave that restaurant feeling light.... ... ... You feel energetic.... ... ... You are in control, and it feels effortless.

I am now going to ask you to imagine something else.... ... ... Because you feel so powerful ... ... so motivated and in control ... ... you are beginning to realize that exercising is going to help you lose weight even faster.... ... ... In the past, perhaps you said to yourself, "Exercising is too difficult," or "I don't have the time to exercise," or "I just don't have the energy to exercise." Your subconscious now realizes that this is nonsense.... ... ...

You change your attitude toward exercise right now.... ... ... You bring forth right now all of the positive things that exercise will give you: ... better health ... increased stamina ... discipline ... and weight loss. The list is endless. Bring all of this to the forefront of your mind and leave it there to stay.... ... ... Exercising is now easy for you ... ... you think about it constantly ... ... and you crave it.... ... It is something that you now desire ... ... and your mind accepts this....

You are eliminating all of the negative excuses and focusing on all of the positives. Imagine yourself and how you want to look.... ... See yourself as thin, slim, and in shape. It feels good to automatically be in control. Exercising for you is now just another part of your day, like showering or brushing your teeth are a part of your day. See yourself as thin, in complete control, and feeling more energetic than ever before. You feel wonderful in every way and no excuse or negative perception about exercise will surface. All negative perceptions have been crushed and eliminated. Feel the positive reasons that surround exercise and bring them to the forefront of your mind right now.... Feel it.... Be it.... You are in charge.... You feel good, and nothing challenges these positive feelings. As a result, you will find yourself making the time to exercise and do what is good for you. You will lose weight and maintain it easily. Nothing gets in your way.... You feel energetic.... You enjoy watching the pounds melt away.... You enjoy feeling motivated and envied.

Your subconscious accepts all these suggestions and your reward will be weight loss. It will feel easy and automatic. Exercising is now just another part of your day.

And your inner subconscious now allows the conscious mind to start becoming more aware of the normal sounds around you, the sounds in the room, the sound of my voice, and the sensations in the arms, legs, or the rest of the body. Paying attention to the thoughts and feelings as the conscious mind begins to drift up and return ... And the conscious wakeful awareness returns completely **now** ... right up to the surface of wakefulness ... completely refreshed and alert. Even as the mind drifts up completely now and the eyes are opening **now**.... That's right, eyes open, and wakeful awareness returns completely **now**.

Session 3: Strengthening Your New Skills
CD TRACK 8

Close your eyes and take a nice relaxing deep breath. Breathe in through your nostrils and exhale through your mouth.... Take another deep breath and do the same thing again....

As you continue to relax with the eyes closed, you can begin to recall the experiences that you've already had with hypnosis ... how it felt to focus your attention on your breathing ... remembering the voice speaking to you and the words from that voice.... As you began to drift down ... very quickly ... very effortlessly ... remembering those feelings in your body ... those feelings of relaxation perhaps ... those heavy feelings or those light feelings ... the sensations in your fingers or toes perhaps ... and what your mind was saying to you as you began to enter that deep hypnotic state ... the images and sensations that came to mind ... that altered feeling in awareness ... as your conscious mind drifted elsewhere and your subconscious mind became more and more active ... more and more quickly ... that's right ... actively guiding and directing your thoughts and your responses ... remembering how your body touched the chair ... remembering the position you were in ... and what was said to you ... and how you felt as you easily allowed that trance to continue.

As you continue to re-experience those feelings ... those sensations ... the memories of those events ... enjoy giving yourself the opportunity to allow that relaxing, drifting state to continue ... as you allow yourself to effortlessly drift deeper and deeper into a state of relaxation.

The interesting thing about Power Programming the mind is that the free-floating sensation can make you overlook certain things you are feeling.... ... ... Now, I am going to ask you to imagine certain feelings.... You don't know what those feelings are yet but as soon as I direct your attention to them, you will pay complete attention to those sensations and go even deeper....

Simply because I say so and for no other reason, all of your attention suddenly goes to the feeling of your hands touching against your thighs or armrest ... and you go deeper....

Now, because I say so and for no other reason, all of your attention suddenly focuses on your pants touching your leg.... And you go deeper.... Now your attention goes to the feeling of the chair, or the surface where you are sitting or lying, pressing up against your back.... And you go deeper.... The next time you do this kind of relaxation, all you have to do is bring your attention to this feeling of the something pressing against your back and you will instantly reach this same deep state.

When I was a child I was told that I had to finish everything on my plate, even if I was full.... ... ... and that message stayed with me for many years.... ... ... My mind was programmed to react that way and I felt sorry for all the poor people in the world.... ... ... Chances are, you too were told to clean your plate.... ... ...

Eventually I realized how silly it was to punish my body and jeopardize my health because of things I had no control over, and I decided to re-program my mind in an opposite way.... ... ...

Now, I simply close my eyes and allow myself to relax the same way you are so relaxed at this very moment.... ... ... I imagine myself at the dinner table feeling quite comfortable leaving food on my plate ... ... just as you have been doing. Your subconscious mind is providing you with the exact same messages as mine, so you are always in control of what you eat.... ... ...

Imagine a smile on your face.... ... ... You have freed yourself from your cravings and compulsions.... ... ... You have freed yourself from overeating ... and you do it effortlessly.... ... ... Certainly our parents didn't mean any harm telling us to eat everything on our plate.... ... ... They came from a different generation when food wasn't abundant.... ... ... But it is abundant now, in fact, too abundant.... ... ... You are beginning to realize now that you never will run out of food ... ... that your portion sizes are always sensible ... ... and that you are through overeating.... ... ... You are done with it for good and your mind accepts this message.... ... ...

Your subconscious is now free from cravings, compulsions, and overeating and you never want to feel full again.... ... ... You now feel obligated to leave food on your plate ... ... and you do it easily.... ... ... You are not a food storage bin.... ... ... You are a human and all humans love to have control of themselves.... ... ... So I'm suggesting to your subconscious that you always demonstrate self-control easily and effortlessly by eating less and always being in control.... ... ... You always eat slowly.... ... ... You always notice when hunger disappears ... ... and you stop eating, and that feels ok. That feels normal.... ... ... That feels good.... ... ...

Imagine now that there is a plate in front of you, overflowing with all of your favorite foods, and you leave a lot of it on the plate easily and effortlessly. And that feels good, that feels normal.... ... ... That's what we are supposed to do.... ... ... You are no longer obligated to eat everything on your plate or to feel guilty for throwing food away.... ... ... You are not a waste can.... ... ... You are a self-controlled individual, and that feels good.... ... ... Your subconscious will provide you with evidence of how true this is.... ... ... Feel how good it is to have control of your life.... ... ... Feel it.... ... ... It is okay....

From this point on, you always leave food on your plate ... ... and your mind accepts this.... ... ... You are always motivated and in control.... ... ... And that same motivation and self-control drives you to exercise on a regular basis.... ... ...

You have every right to feel good about yourself.... ... ... You feel liberated.... ... ... You feel free from your past habits and compulsions ... ... and nothing stops you from achieving your weight loss goal.... ... ...

See an image of yourself six months from now, looking exactly how you want to look.... ... ... Your mind is now fueled to make this a reality.... ... ... And

nothing stops you ... ... nothing stops you.... ... ... This is your reality now....
... ... This is the new you.... ... ...

I am now going to count from 1 to 5. And when I reach the number 5,
you will open your eyes fully, feeling completely refreshed and alert.... 1 ...
coming out of that deep trance state, feeling wonderful in every way, feeling
completely confident and in control in every way ... 2 ... continuing to emerge
now, feeling wonderful in every way ... 3 ... starting to come back now ... 4 ...
eyes are starting to open ... and 5 ... eyes are now wide open, and you are
feeling refreshed and alert and wonderful in every way.

HOW TO RECORD YOUR OWN POWER PROGRAMMING SESSIONS

As you continue to work with Power Programming, one very effective way to keep the process fresh and fine-tuned is to record your own customized Power Programming sessions. That way, you can tailor scripts to your own individual goals and needs. Some people respond better to someone else's voice instead of their own. If that's true of you, you might want to ask another person to do the recording for you.

Each session should take about 20 minutes to record. It's best to record the entire session in one sitting. Speak slowly and clearly in a smooth and relaxed tone of voice, and make sure your voice is somewhat monotone and calm. In the script that follows, wherever you see ellipsis points (a series of dots) you should pause for a moment. The more dots you see, the longer you should pause. Listen carefully to your Power Programming CD to get a better idea of the speaking voice and style that is most effective. Also, you might want to play soft classical music in the background to help yourself relax. Make sure that there are no distractions while you listen to your session, such as kids screaming, cell phones ringing, or dogs barking.

Here are two Power Programming sessions for you to record on your own. You can alter the words however you wish, in order to make them more effective for your individual situation.

PERSONALIZED POWER PROGRAMMING

Session 1

Step 1: Relaxation

You are about to have a very stimulating and rewarding experience. Use your vivid imagination in a very active way to help yourself achieve the results you desire....

Take a deep breath through your nostrils very slowly ... that's right.... Let the air out very slowly through your mouth.... Take another deep breath, through your nostrils ... and let the air out very slowly through your mouth.... Each time you breathe from this point forward, imagine that your breath is flowing freely through your entire body, spreading total relaxation.... Feel the relaxation now.... ... ...

Your imagination is a very valuable tool.... During the course of this session, you will imagine certain things.... There is no right or wrong way for you to direct your mind.... Imagine a green beach, for example, and most likely you can imagine that beach now even though there is probably no green beach anywhere in the world.... Your subconscious does not discriminate.... You can imagine anything you want to, and your mind will accept it....

Imagine a white ball of light up above in the sky of your mind.... Perhaps you can see it in your mind.... Maybe you can feel it or hear it.... Whichever way you imagine it is perfectly fine.... Imagine that white light as a wonderful, relaxing, soothing light.... This white light has very powerful and healing properties ... properties that are going to allow you to relax every muscle and every cell in your entire body ... from the top of your head to the tips of your toes.... Begin to feel that relaxation.... Now, imagine that this white light is coming down very slowly from the sky and it enters your body through the top of your scalp.... Perhaps you can feel it as it begins to melt into your entire facial area, spreading total relaxation.... You can feel your entire facial area beginning to relax already.... You can feel it spreading slowly and peacefully throughout your face....

Focus your attention on your forehead now and allow your forehead to relax.... Feel your forehead beginning to relax.... Relax your eyebrows now ...

and your cheeks.... Relax your nose and your mouth ... and especially all of those tiny muscles around your mouth and lips.... Starting ... to relax.... Make sure that your teeth are parted just a little bit.... Just relax.... Wonderful....

The relaxation from this wonderful, soothing light is beginning to make its way to your neck now and your neck is beginning to relax ... the front part of your neck ... and the back part of your neck ... right through to your shoulders.... Feel your shoulders beginning to relax ... that's right.... Get rid of any stress ... tension ... or anxiety that may be in your shoulders or neck area.... This is a place where stress and tension gathers, so make sure to just let it go and relax.... Relaxation makes its way to your arms now and your arms begin to relax ... your upper arms ... your elbows.... Relax your forearms.... Relax your wrists ... and your hands ... and even your fingers. Each and every finger can now completely relax as you begin to drift into a very deep and relaxed state.... Just letting go....

Now just imagine that your arms are becoming very, very heavy ... very loose ... very limp ... and very heavy ... almost as if someone has placed two sand bags on your arms.... So relaxed ... so very heavy....

Just allow yourself to continue to breathe so comfortably and notice how deep and regular your breathing has become.... Feel your breathing ... feel the pace and rhythm of your breathing.... Notice the expansion and contraction of your diaphragm and chest ... and allow all of your chest muscles to relax completely ... all the way down ... slowly to your stomach area.... Feel your stomach muscles as they begin to relax completely.... Get rid of any stress, any tension, any anxiety that may be in your stomach area.... It feels wonderful to just let go and relax.... Nothing to do but relax....

That wonderful relaxation wraps its way around your body now towards your back and your back begins to relax.... The large muscles in your upper back becomes soft and pliable.... The relaxation flows down your spine like a gentle river and into your lower back.... Just relax.... And now your hips are relaxed and especially your legs.... Relax your thighs.... Relax your knees and your calf muscles.... Relax your feet ... and even your toes.... Each and every toe is now completely relaxed.... Just continue to allow all of these muscle groups to relax with each breath you take ... feeling so good and so completely relaxed.

You might experience certain feelings as you drift into this relaxed state.... Your hands or feet, or your arms or legs might feel numb or tingly.... You might feel both a numbness and a tingling sensation....

You might feel either a lightness or a heaviness.... If you have a light feeling, you might feel as if you're just floating above your chair, barely able to feel your body touching it.... If you have a heavy feeling, you might feel as if you're just sinking into the couch or chair, so deeply, with sagging shoulders....

You might feel the need to swallow ... and if you have the need to swallow it is okay to do so.... Or you might feel your eyelids flickering and fluttering very lightly ... that's right....

If you're experiencing any of these feelings, you're ready to allow yourself to enter your subconscious.... It is very gradual and in a few moments you're going to count backwards from 10 to 1, and as you do, you can allow yourself to enter your subconscious at your own pace.... But before you begin to count, use that powerful imagination of yours again.... Now just imagine a soft, cuddly cloud.... The cloud can be any color you choose.... This is the most comfortable cloud in the whole world.... This cloud is going to take you to a very special place in your life.... It can be a real place or an imagined place ... any place you choose ... a place where you're happy, confident, motivated, safe, and secure.... Just allow this soft, relaxing cloud to take you to that very special place.... And as you're counting, you will go deeper and deeper into your subconscious....

Step 2: Going Deeper

And just continue to drift off to that soothing comfortable place as you count from 10 to 1.... And as you count, you will go deeper and deeper into that place....

10 ... going deeper and deeper now ... 9 ... just drifting and relaxing ... 8 ... 7 ... deeper and deeper ... 6 ... just ... letting ... go.... Now ... 5 ... 4 ... all the way down deep ... 3 ... 2 ... and finally ... 1.... Deep ... deep ... deep into your subconscious....

Your mind is now relaxed and completely open to all of the beneficial suggestions that you are about to hear.

Step 3: Imagery

Now that you are so completely relaxed, your subconscious can provide you with very powerful images. Snacking has been a problem for you merely because of perception. Your mind has been exposed for too long to images of sitting in front of the television and craving junk. The truth is, snacking is not really rewarding. This is only a matter of perception. You're going to change this perception and you're going to have complete control and you're going to feel healthy.

Imagine that it is late in the evening now. Perhaps it is eight o'clock, nine o'clock, ten o'clock. It is the time of night when you would normally indulge in a bowl of ice cream or a bag of chips. But things are different this partic-ular night. This particular night it feels just fine to relax without having a snack. It feels okay not having the snack. In fact, the thought of snacking seems very distant. It seems unappealing to you. You realize that this particular night, freedom has become a new part of you, freedom from being a prisoner to intense cravings and desires for junk food. You know that there is ice cream in the freezer and junk food in the kitchen cabinets. But tonight, you find that you easily and effortlessly reject them. The very thought of them turns you off. The thought of nurturing and rewarding yourself in this way seems very important to you.

From this point on, you will snack on food only when you are hungry, and at no other time. Your subconscious mind is accepting this suggestion fully, and when you are hungry you desire healthy snacks, such as fruits or gra-nola bars.

Imagine that you are sitting on your couch now. The comfort and relax-ation of your body absorbing into that soft couch is rewarding enough for you. You appreciate this kind of relaxation after a long day. And as you relax on your couch, imagine that you have a slight hunger feeling. You know there is fresh, ripe fruit in the refrigerator and your thoughts become very attracted to that fruit. Imagine getting up from the couch now and walking into the kitchen. Perhaps you go into the cabinet and get out a bowl or a plate to place the mouth-watering fruit on. You make your way over to the refrigera-tor to get that fruit. Your mind is attracted toward the fruit like a magnet, and you immediately smell fruit when you open the refrigerator. You salivate just thinking about the healthy, delicious fruit that will satisfy your slight hunger. The thought of fattening junk food is extremely unappetizing. You reject fattening snacks and you do it automatically and effortlessly. It feels wonderful having this kind of automatic control. Feel that control now ... feel it....

Now, imagine that you are taking a bite of that fruit. Feel the texture as you sink your teeth into it. The cool juices from the fruit fill your entire mouth, stimulating your taste buds like never before. And as you swallow, you can feel the coolness, the cleanness, the healthfulness of that fruit as it slowly glides down your throat and into your stomach, like a healthy child gliding down a waterslide in a water park.

From this moment on, your craving for snack foods ceases to exist. You find yourself having light, healthy snacks only when you feel hungry and at no other time. You easily and effortlessly resist the fattening junk snacks and select the healthful fruit snacks. You do this easily, automatically and effortlessly. Your subconscious mind accepts these suggestions. By eating healthfully and enjoying it, you reward yourself when you're hungry. It is your new normality. Snacking is simply eliminated from your being. You never feel bored when you're in control of your actions.

Step 4: Forceful Commands

Today you have begun a positive approach to attaining a new slim, healthy, and attractive body. The following suggestions are going to be fully accepted by your subconscious mind, allowing you to make permanent positive changes in your eating habits. These suggestions are going to become a permanent part of your everyday life, giving you a new sense of normalcy. You are going to be quite surprised by the effectiveness of these suggestions. Your entire approach, feelings, and desires toward food and eating are going to be recreated, giving you new, easy, and normal methods for losing weight.

Your new approach toward eating is going to allow you to eat the way nature intended. You will enjoy food and eat food in a positive, healthful manner. In fact, you are going to enjoy eating in a healthful, controlled way much more than that old uncontrolled way. From now on, you thrive on the fact that you are going to eat all that you need physiologically and that you will be completely satisfied doing so. Your appetite will now be your pal. You will listen very attentively to your appetite and pay very close attention to it. You will realize how normal it is to eat when you're hungry and only when you're hungry. You realize that eating when you're not hungry is unnecessary and that you will never need to do that again.

Because you have made your appetite your buddy, you will start paying attention to it much more while you're in the process of eating, too. When you are eating in a very slow and enjoyable fashion, you will stop as soon as the hunger feeling disappears. In the past, perhaps you were eating until you became full. When you pay attention to your appetite and your appetite becomes your friend, you stop long before you're full. You stop when the hunger feeling first goes away and you feel satisfied doing this. It is okay. It feels just fine doing this. You will never again need to feel full in order to feel satisfied. Feeling full makes you bloated and fat. Feeling full makes you feel out of control. You will never want to feel full again.

In the past, you didn't pay attention to your appetite at all because you were eating emotionally. Emotions create cravings, urges, and obsessions about food. You think that eating will help you feel better. This is far from the truth. Eating too much when it is unnecessary actually increases negative emotions. Because you have made a friend of your appetite, you will eat only when you have hunger and at no other time. You will feel just fine doing this and you will do it easily and effortlessly. You have begun to pay such close attention to your appetite that you will know when you've had enough and you will feel comfortable stopping when you've had enough. You will never want to feel full again. You will never need to crave food again when you're not hungry. You have learned to tune into your new appetite, your buddy, and if you eat too much against your buddy's advice, you will have violated your normal reflexes.

Now, imagine yourself as you want to look—slim, attractive, and healthy. Learning to pay attention to your normal body reflexes will make eating sensibly simple to do. Being overweight is not a dietary problem. It is an emotional problem. You are eliminating the notion that food makes you feel good. Eating normally when you're hungry, and being in control of how much food you eat makes you feel good. It demonstrates that you have taken control of your life. You are simply forming a new habit to eat only when you feel hunger and to stop as soon as the hunger goes away. You are going to be slim and attractive. You will feel fantastic and in control all over. Dieting, cravings, and compulsions are all removed from your mind now. You are simply bringing back your normal reflexes, reflexes that allow you to be in control of your eating and identify your hunger correctly.

You will prove to your own satisfaction just how in control you are as a human being by paying attention to the following suggestion and allowing your subconscious mind to fully accept and actualize it: From now on, any time you feel even the slightest craving or temptation to eat anything that you know is wrong for you or to eat any time that you are not hungry, you will say "no way" and easily stick by it because the rewards of being in control and becoming slimmer are far more important to you than eating an unhealthy diet.

Step 5: Returning to Your Conscious State

I am now going to count from 1 to 5 and when I reach the number 5, you will open your eyes fully, feeling completely refreshed and alert ... 1 ... coming out of that deep state, feeling wonderful in every way, feeling completely confident and in control in every way ... 2 ... continuing to emerge now, feeling wonderful in every way ... 3 ... starting to come back now ... 4 ... eyes are starting to open ... and 5 ... eyes are now wide open, and you're feeling refreshed and alert and wonderful in every way.

PERSONALIZED POWER PROGRAMMING

Session 2

Step 1: Relaxation

Make sure that you are sitting or lying down in a comfortable position. Find a small object, preferably something that is shiny. Fix your eyes on that object and don't take your eyes off of it.... Take a few deep breaths now.... Just keep breathing deeply and listen to the sound of my voice.... As you continue to fix your eyes on the object, you will find that your eyelids have a tendency to get heavy ... almost as if a heavy weight has been attached to them ... and the longer you stare at this object, the more your eyelids get heavy ... and you blink, and your eyelids feel like something is pulling them down, as if they want to slowly close.... Your eyelids get sleepier and heavier now ... and you feel them slowly closing ... slowly closing ... getting drowsier and more tired.... And when they finally close, you feel so good ... drowsy, heavy feeling ... pulling down ... down ... down ... slowly closing.... The harder you try, the harder it is to keep them open.... You feel that very soon they will close tightly ... almost closing now ... that's right ... almost tightly closing now.... Your eyes are tightly closed.... You feel wonderful.... You feel comfortable.... You are completely relaxed now.... Just let yourself drift and enjoy this comfortable relaxed state.... You will find that your entire body feels heavier now ... heavier ... and you just drift into a deeply relaxed state....

Step 2: Going Deeper

And it's interesting as you relax so completely ... it's interesting that you are experiencing certain feelings now that you are not even aware of.... But the moment I bring your attention to one of those feelings, you instantly become aware of it ... and you go even deeper the moment I mention it....

One feeling that you are experiencing right now but are not aware of—but you will be aware of the moment I say it—is the feeling of your chest expanding as you breathe ... and you go deeper....

Now, another feeling that you are feeling but are not aware of right now—but will be the moment I bring it to your attention—is the feeling of your eyeballs moving in your eye sockets ... and you go even deeper....

Now, I'm going to bring your attention to a feeling that you are going to be super aware of the moment I mention it ... and that is the feeling of relaxation taking place all over your body ... and you go even deeper now and you are completely and totally relaxed....

Step 3: Imagery

Right now, whether you realize it or not, your mind and body are completely relaxed, and your mind is completely open and receptive to every image and suggestion that I'm about to give you.... First of all, you are here, listening, because you want to be ... because you truly want to lose weight.... And you are going to lose weight and you are going to do it easily and effortlessly.... You're going to imagine some pretty powerful things right now.... Just know that your mind is going to be completely receptive to these images and you are going to find yourself responding to these images every day....

Imagine that it is Monday morning, you have just awakened and are ready to begin your day.... Imagine stretching out your arms and taking a refreshing breath of air.... It is a beautiful day outside and you feel well-rested and ready to begin your day.... It is now time to eat breakfast and you find yourself desiring a healthy breakfast like cereal or fruit.... You sit down to eat and find that you thoroughly enjoy eating your healthy, hearty breakfast.... The thought of fattening, greasy bacon and eggs completely turns you off.... It makes you think of growing fat.... You easily avoid those kinds of breakfast foods.... You finish your breakfast now and are ready to head out.... You feel wonderful and energized....

It is later in the morning now and you feel a slight bit of hunger.... Thankfully, you are prepared.... You take out a juicy, fresh piece of fruit and you sink your teeth into it, enjoying it like never before.... Imagine the juices of that fruit tickling your taste buds.... It tastes so delicious and completely satisfies you.... You feel so in control....

Now it is lunchtime and that feeling of self-control stays with you.... Again, you are prepared for lunch.... You look forward to a healthy lunch and find it effortless to avoid unhealthy lunches.... Imagine sitting down and eating a healthy grilled chicken or turkey sandwich or a fresh, healthy salad.... These are the kinds of foods you crave for lunch now.... Fast food, roast beef sandwiches, pizza, and hoagies completely turn you off.... You don't want them.... You don't need them.... You enjoy eating healthfully and feeling in control.... You are always in control from now on and it feels wonderful....

Now it is dinnertime.... Again, you have a wonderful feeling of self-control.... You sit down and eat your healthy meal and you find yourself eating slowly and leaving food on your plate.... It's easy for you to eat slowly and leave food on your plate.... This is what you crave from now on: ... pure self-control....

Step 4: Forceful Commands

Now that you know what it feels like to be in control, you are going to find it easy to do, no matter where you are.... From now on, you crave healthy foods like fruits and vegetables and lean meats.... You find it effortless to avoid junk food and snacking.... From now on, whenever you feel like having a snack, the first thing that is going to come to your mind is your favorite fruit ... and that is going to satisfy you completely.... Your mind accepts this command.... You find it easy and effortless to avoid ice cream, cookies, and cakes.... You find them unappealing.... You find them unnecessary.... You dislike them ... and your mind accepts this.... From now on, every time you sit down for a meal, you find yourself eating something that is healthy and you find yourself eating slowly.... You eat slowly from now on.... You pay attention to your hunger feeling and you stop eating long before you are full.... That's right, you stop eating long before you're full every time you eat ... and this further elevates your confidence and self-control.... You are always in control and your mind accepts this command.... For you, it is easy to be in control.... It is easy to avoid unhealthy snacks and desserts.... It is easy to leave food on your plate ... and ... it is easy to lose weight.... You are always in control ... and your mind accepts all of these commands....

Step 5: Returning to Your Conscious State

I am now going to count from 1 to 5 and when I reach the number 5 you will open your eyes fully, feeling completely refreshed and alert ... 1 ... coming out of that deep state, feeling wonderful in every way, feeling completely confident and in control in every way ... 2 ... continuing to emerge now, feeling wonderful in every way ... 3 ... starting to come back now ... 4 ... eyes are starting to open ... and 5 ... eyes are now wide open, and you're feeling refreshed and alert and wonderful in every way.

A Final Word

When I look into people's eyes and see doubt, fear, frustration, and guilt, and then watch them transform themselves into confident people who are in control of their lives, I'm always excited by the incredible power we all have to change ourselves and our behavior. You can make the same kind of transformation, and that's why I wrote this book.

Several years ago, I received a call from a frantic mother who was desperate for help. Her twelve-year-old son, Timmy, had the unusual habit of putting his entire fist in his mouth and sucking on it constantly. You might be wondering how he could have fit his entire fist in his mouth, but, trust me, this boy did it all the time. After talking with Timmy's mom for a little while over the phone, I arranged to meet her and her son.

When Timmy and his mom came into my office, I realized how serious the problem was. This poor boy did practically everything with his fist in his mouth. He did his homework, played video games, and even drank with his fist in his mouth. What upset me most was the fact that the teeth on the left side of Timmy's mouth had been unable to grow in normally, because his fist was always in the way.

Timmy's mom had tried everything to help her son. She had taken him to top doctors who even put him on medication, but nothing worked. She heard about me from a friend who used Power Programming to stop biting her fingernails and, although she was skeptical, she decided that she had nothing to lose. Although I had never worked with this particular problem before, I realized that it came directly from Timmy's subconscious mind and it could be eliminated using Power Programming.

Timmy and I talked about his habit for a few minutes, and then I used the Power Programming method with him. Forty-five minutes later, his hand sucking was gone—and it never came back. Timmy's mother was amazed and extremely grateful, but I pointed out to her that I didn't cure Timmy. *He did.* I didn't have special powers over his mind; I simply helped him direct his mind to the right place. If Power Programming could so quickly and easily help someone stop an unusual habit like this one, you know that it can help you change your eating and exercise habits!

We all come equipped with a supercomputer right on top of our shoulders. The control center for this computer is your subconscious mind, and as you now know, it is responsible for everything you do. But, unfortunately, it doesn't come with a written instruction manual. Please look at this book-with-CD program as a handbook for accessing your subconscious, knowing that the magic of your mind can eliminate any harmful or destructive behavior patterns from your life. Always remember that you have full control over your own life. You have the power to achieve any goal, no matter how impossible it may seem.

Enjoy the new you!

Index

About the Author

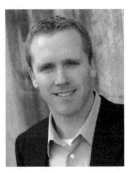

TOM KERSTING, LPC, PH.D. was a successful college baseball pitcher when a slump in his performance threatened to derail him. Fortunately, a teammate referred him to a doctor who taught him how to use mental techniques to successfully revive his pitching ability. It worked so well that, after playing in college and semi-professionally, he shifted his career path from baseball to psychology, counseling, and hypnotherapy.

Later in life, when Dr. Kersting began to gain excess weight, he returned to the mental approach that had salvaged his baseball career. Again, he was so successful, he went on to develop the *Power Programming* weight loss method that has since helped thousands at his Westwood, New Jersey, weight loss clinic.

Dr. Kersting holds advanced degrees in counseling, human development, and hypnotherapy. He is a seasoned speaker and has lectured extensively in the greater New York City area, stimulating and motivating audiences with his charisma, passion, and enthusiasm.

Dr. Kersting publishes a very successful biweekly e-newsletter, available through his website, www.losingweightwhendietsfail.com. He lives with his wife and two children in Upper Saddle River, New Jersey.